Screening in
Chronic Disease

Monographs in Epidemiology and Biostatistics

edited by Jennifer L. Kelsey, Michael G. Marmot, Paul D. Stolley, Martin P. Vessey

MONOGRAPHS IN EPIDEMIOLOGY AND BIOSTATISTICS
VOLUME 19

Screening in Chronic Disease

Second Edition

ALAN S. MORRISON

New York   Oxford
OXFORD UNIVERSITY PRESS
1992

93-347

Oxford University Press

Oxford   New York   Toronto
Delhi   Bombay   Calcutta   Madras   Karachi
Kuala Lumpur   Singapore   Hong Kong   Tokyo
Nairobi   Dar es Salaam   Cape Town
Melbourne   Auckland   Madrid

and associated companies in
Berlin   Ibadan

Copyright © 1985, 1992 by Oxford University Press, Inc.

Published by Oxford University Press, Inc.
200 Madison Avenue, New York, New York 10016

Oxford is a registered trademark of Oxford University Press

Library of Congress Cataloging-in-Publication Data
Morrison, Alan S.
Screening in chronic disease / Alan S. Morrison.—2nd ed.
p. cm.   (Monographs in epidemiology and biostatistics ; v. 19)
Includes bibliographical references and index.
ISBN 0-19-506390-2
1. Chronic diseases—Diagnosis.
2. Chronic diseases—Epidemiology.
3. Medical screening—Methodology.
I. Title.   II. Series.
[DNLM: 1. Chronic Disease.   2. Epidemiologic Methods.
3. Evaluation Studies.   4. Preventive Health Services.
W1 M0567LT v. 19 / WA 245 M878s]
RA644.5.M67   1992   362.1'77–dc20   DNLM/DLC
for Library of Congress
91-32429

The following tables include copyrighted material that was reproduced with permission:

Tables 3–1, 6–4, and 7–3. From Farrow GM: Pathologist's role in bladder cancer.
Semin Oncol 1978; 6:198–206. Reprinted by permission of Grune & Stratton, Inc.

Table 7–4. From Morrison AS: Public health value of using epidemiologic information
to identify high-risk groups for bladder cancer screening. *Semin Oncol* 1979; 6:184–188.
Reprinted by permission of Grune & Stratton, Inc.

Table 8–1. From Foster RS Jr, Lang SP, Costanza MC, Worden JK, Haines CR, Yates JW:
Breast self-examination practices and breast-cancer stage. *N Engl J Med* 1978; 299:265–270.
Reprinted by permission of the New England Journal of Medicine.

9   8   7   6   5   4   3   2   1

Printed in the United States of America
on acid-free paper

Foreword

Alan Morrison died of cancer on May 17, 1992, at the age of 49. When that happened, the world lost one of its best epidemiologists, and I lost one of my best friends. Alan was someone you could count on to look out for your well-being, to put you first and himself second. You also could count on him to give independent thought to any issue, and to express that thought in a coherent and—even if he disagreed with *your* thought on the issue—in a kind way. Alan was totally without pretense. He had a great sense of humor and, likely as not, he served as the butt of his own joke or anecdote. It was always fun to be around him.

While he made a number of important contributions to our understanding of disease etiology, Alan is best known for his work on the principles of early detection of cancer and other chronic diseases. After writing several influential journal articles on the subject, in 1985 he published the first edition of his book, *Screening in Chronic Disease*. The present edition, completed just before his death, retains the best features of the original. For example, the first chapter was written either to stand on its own as an overview of the principles of screening, or as an introduction to the topics covered in the remainder of the book. Chapter 4, devoted to experimental studies, brings the relevant issues to life by considering in depth one such study (the HIP trial of breast cancer screening), yet manages to cover the subject in general terms as well. The description of healthy screenee bias in Chapter 5, supplemented by descriptions of some research settings in which it has been present, should prove just as instructive to readers in the 1990s as it was to their counterparts one decade earlier.

New to this edition are, among other things, a greater level of detail on the analysis of nonexperimental studies of screening efficacy and of "intermediate" endpoints. New chapters, the final three, have been devoted to a review of available data pertaining to the efficacy of screening for breast and cervical cancers and for risk factors for arteriosclerotic vascular disease. These chapters make an important contribution to the book as a whole, in that they allow the reader to

1. see the ways in which the research methods described earlier in the book can be applied to specific issues in screening,
2. appreciate the roles and relative contributions of different types of design in arriving at inferences regarding screening efficacy,
3. understand what is the current basis for recommending (or not recommending) screening for these conditions, and what additional research would be useful to conduct.

Alan's economical but thorough style of writing, as well as his consistently balanced interpretations, characterize the present edition as they did the original.

Given society's ever-increasing concern with health care costs, ever-increasing attention is being paid to the amount of benefit we receive for expenditures devoted to health. Screening activities will no doubt be scrutinized with particular care, given their potential for generating large aggregate costs. Thus, a book such as this one—a book that lays a foundation for estimating the presence and magnitude of health benefits associated with screening, and for judging a cost-effective interval between screens—should be a useful resource for some time to come.

In the preface to the first edition, Alan stated that the effects of screening "are usually not observable in individuals. An important goal of the book is to show that these effects can be understood by appropriate comparisons of *groups*." Many teachers and writers of the principles of epidemiology have tried to show that the effects of *etiologic* factors can be understood by appropriate comparisons of groups. However, most of us shied away from any broad attempt to understand, much less describe, what "appropriate comparisons" mean in the context of screening. It took Alan Morrison to weave together for us a coherent whole, and in so doing also illuminate individual parts of that whole which hadn't before been seen. Our debt to him can now only be repaid by continued development of the principles and methods he has set forth, and by the application of these principles and methods to gauge correctly the impact of a given screening test.

Noel S. Weiss

Preface

The focus of this second edition, as with the first, is measurement of the effects of early detection and treatment on the natural history of disease, and evaluation of the usefulness of screening in reducing morbidity and mortality. The primary goals of the revision were to improve the presentations of methods of analysis of follow-up and case-control studies and of the use of determinants of outcome (early outcomes) in predicting the results of screening, and to add chapters on screening for cancer of the breast, cardiovascular disease, and cancer of the cervix.

The avoidance of healthy-screenee bias has proven to be a challenging issue in the analysis of nonexperimental studies of the value of screening, especially case-control studies. The approach that I described in the first edition of this book was unnecessarily restrictive. I have now outlined a method of analysis that I hope is more satisfying. Dr. Dana Flanders pointed out to me that the limitations of my earlier approach were avoidable (see Flanders and Longini, 1990). I am grateful to Dr. Flanders and to Dr. Nicholas Lange for their advice on this topic.

The HIP study of screening for breast cancer (Shapiro et al, 1988) has continued to occupy a central position in this field. The HIP investigators and Dr. Philip Prorok, Early Detection Branch, National Cancer Institute, kindly gave me access to data from the HIP study. I have drawn on this material for examples of the analysis of both experimental and nonexperimental studies, and the use of determinants of outcome, and I have revised earlier, incomplete, analyses of lead time, lead time bias, and length bias in the HIP study.

In the last few years, researchers, public health workers, and medical practitioners have been faced with a steady stream of reports on screening for chronic diseases. Much of this information concerns breast cancer, cardiovascular disease, or cervical cancer. Each of these diseases is an important scientific and public health problem. Each has been the object of a number of investigations, but the methods used to study each of these diseases have differed substantially from the methods used to study the others. The three chapters on these diseases concern the value of early treatment in the context of screening with presently available tests. Together these reviews illustrate many problems of design, analysis, and interpretation. They also serve to emphasize the challenges of deriving practical and rewarding screening policies from research results. I have included detailed summaries of the studies that I reviewed so that readers will have at hand the information on which the interpretations and conclusions are based.

I prepared much of the second edition while I was on sabbatical leave from Brown University. I thank Prof. Nicholas Wald and his colleagues at the Department of Environmental and Preventive Medicine, Medical College of St. Bartholomew's Hospital, London, for their hospitality during that period. I benefited from discussions with Prof. Wald and Drs. Howard Cuckle, Christopher Frost, and Malcolm Law, and I thank Dr. Law for his comments on the chapter on cervical cancer. The study in Jack Mongar and Carol MacCormack's mews house was delightful.

Diana Anderson, RN, Joyce Babcock, and Susan Waterman were instrumental in preparing the manuscript for publication. Their efforts were directed by Wendy Verhoek-Oftedahl, Ph.D. whose assistance in this project has been significant.

Dr. Jacques Brisson offered his comments on various aspects of this book. I deeply appreciate Dr. Brisson's continuing collaboration. I am indebted to Jeffrey House and the editorial staff at Oxford University Press for their guidance and encouragement in the preparation of both editions.

Providence, R.I.   A.S.M.
December 1991

Preface to the
First Edition

Screening asymptomatic people to detect and treat chronic diseases early
has become an important part of medicine and public health. Yet, sufficient information is not available on whether most screening procedures
are worthwhile, or on how often, and to whom, they should be applied.
This volume presents methods for investigating such problems. I hope that
it will be useful in courses that contain material on principles of screening
or on the epidemiology and control of cancer and other chronic diseases,
and that it will also serve as a reference for the design, analysis, and interpretation of studies on screening.

The focus of this book is the description and measurement of changes
in the natural history of disease that are brought about by early detection
and treatment. These changes are the result of lead time, the prolongation
of life of cases treated early, and prognostic selection (including "length
bias"). Screening may appear difficult to understand because its effects are
usually not observable in individuals. An important goal of the book is to
show that these effects can be understood by appropriate comparisons of
groups.

The presentation is based on relationships between the natural history
of disease and measures of disease frequency. Chapter 1 is a general and
relatively nontechnical summary that introduces much of the terminology
used, providing an orientation to the discussion that follows. This chapter
also is designed as background reading for one to three hours of intro-
ductory lectures on screening that might be part of an elementary epidemiology course for students of medicine or public health. Topics covered
subsequently include the definition and evaluation of test sensitivity; the
measurement of lead time; methods for assessing the extent to which early
treatment reduces morbidity or prolongs life; the effects of treatment, lead
time, and length-biased sampling on the observed prognosis of screen-

detected patients; the evaluation of test specificity and the roles of specificity and high-risk groups in determining the feasibility and costs of screening programs; and issues in setting screening policy, including the use of models. Some basic material on epidemiologic methods integral to the presentation is reviewed in context. This material includes measures of disease frequency and certain aspects of the structure and analysis of experimental studies and nonexperimental follow-up and case-control studies. Recent textbooks by Breslow and Day (1980), Kleinbaum et al (1982), and Schlesselman (1982) give general discussions of epidemiologic methods, including study design, data collection, sources of bias, and procedures for point and interval estimation of exposure-disease relationships.

The illustrations in this book are drawn primarily from cancer-screening programs, since most of the methodologic developments in screening and most studies of its efficacy in disease control have concerned cancer. The study of screening for breast cancer done by investigators at the Health Insurance Plan of Greater New York (HIP) is a uniquely rich source of illustrative material, and I have drawn on it heavily, as have others. However, examples are also taken from screening for nonmalignant diseases such as hypertension and diabetes. The field of disease control through the use of early diagnosis and treatment is developing rapidly, and the acquisition of valid new information is of much more importance than is the reassessment of data already in hand. Therefore, I have not attempted to provide a comprehensive review of the results of screening or a set of screening recommendations. For these purposes readers are referred to documents by the American Cancer Society (1980), a Canadian Task Force (1980), and Miller (1978). The economic cost of screening is a crucial determinant of its usefulness in disease control, but I have dealt with questions of cost in only a very general way. Eddy (1980) and Weinstein and Stason (1976) have considered the cost implications of various screening and treatment policies in detail.

This book began with a paper that Philip Cole and I wrote, entitled "Basic issues in population screening for cancer" (1980). Large parts of Chapter 1, as well as sections of other chapters, are based on that paper. I am indebted to Dr. Cole and to Dr. Brian MacMahon for their support and encouragement in this and other areas of epidemiology over a period of many years. I thank Dr. Jacques Brisson for many perceptive and helpful comments, and Drs. David Eddy, John Emerson, Gary Friedman, George Hutchison, Philip Prorok, Elio Riboli, and Noel Weiss for their advice. Finally, I appreciate the careful, critical reading of drafts of the text by the series editor, Dr. Abraham Lilienfeld, who died on August 6, 1984.

Financial support for this work was provided by a Faculty Research Award (FRA-208) from the American Cancer Society and a Special Projects Grant (1 D04 AH01693) from the Department of Health and Human Services.

Providence, R.I.   A.S.M.
November 1984

Contents

Screening in
Chronic Disease

1 Introduction

Screening for disease control can be defined as the examination of asymptomatic people in order to classify them as likely, or unlikely, to have the disease that is the object of screening. People who appear likely to have the disease are investigated further to arrive at a final diagnosis. Those people who are found to have the disease are then treated. The organized application of early diagnosis and treatment activities in large groups often is described as "mass screening" or "population screening." The goal of screening is to reduce morbidity or mortality from the disease by early treatment of the cases discovered. Screening is an extension of the process by which people perceive symptoms of their own illnesses and then consult physicians for diagnosis and treatment. Screening simply calls attention to the likelihood of disease before symptoms appear.

The use of the word *screening* in connection with early diagnosis and treatment should be distinguished from other uses of the term in epidemiology and medicine. First, screening may refer to a series of tests done on a *symptomatic* patient for whom a diagnosis has not yet been established. Someone who seeks medical care because of blood in the urine may have a urinalysis, urine culture, cystoscopy, bladder biopsy, x-ray examinations, and blood chemistry studies in order to identify the disease causing the bleeding. This type of screening is part of the practice of clinical medicine rather than public health or preventive medicine. Second, chemical agents may be screened by means of laboratory tests or epidemiologic surveillance in order to identify those substances likely to be toxic. Third, screening procedures such as those described in this book may be used to estimate the prevalence of various conditions without immediate disease-control objectives (Bishop et al, 1975; Rogan and Gladen, 1978). Finally, screening sometimes refers to the identification of people at high *risk* of a disease. For example, a program might be devised to find cigarette smokers

3

and help them quit smoking in order to reduce their risk of heart disease and various respiratory ailments. The line between a risk factor and a disease is not sharp. Hypertension can be viewed as either a risk factor for cardiovascular disease or as an early manifestation of it. Polyps of the colon, or dysplasia or carcinoma in situ of the cervix, are equally well considered to be risk factors or diseases. Breast cancer is consistently described as a disease. The long-term goal of screening, however, is to prevent disability or death, not the disease in itself. The presence of asymptomatic breast cancer is certainly a risk factor for those events. All screening with the aim of early treatment involves the identification of asymptomatic persons based on their risk of a serious outcome. For simplicity, the term *disease* is defined as any characteristic of anatomy (eg, cancer or arteriosclerosis), physiology (eg, hypertension or hyperlipidemia), or behavior (eg, smoking) that is associated with an elevated risk of serious illness or death.

Programs of early diagnosis and treatment nearly always are directed at diseases that are not known to be infectious: cancer, diabetes, glaucoma, and so on. The idea that such diseases can be controlled in this way is a phenomenon of the twentieth century. A time-honored means of controlling infectious diseases, however, is to detect cases in order to isolate or treat them. A decree in 1347 directed that prostitutes in Avignon, France, were to be examined weekly for venereal disease to protect their clients (Haggard, 1929). If case finding to control an infectious disease is successful, it is the result of interrupting the transmission of the disease. In contrast, most present-day screening activities are based on the premise that treatment will retard or stop the progression of established cases of disease that are detected early, while later treatment is likely to be less effective.

This modern concept of screening has roots in pathology, clinical medicine, and in public health and vital statistics. Studies of the pathology and cytology of cancer of the cervix have been the source of many fundamental ideas. Epithelial changes in the cervix were described in 1886, and carcinoma in situ was identified in 1908. Exfoliative cytology of the female genital tract dates from the mid-nineteenth century, but not until the late 1920s was it found that cervical cancer cells could be recognized in cytology specimens (Breslow et al, 1979). *Diagnosis of Uterine Cancer by the Vaginal Smear,* by Papanicolaou and Traut, was published in 1943. The work described in that book is the single most important reason for the enormous increase in cancer-screening activities during the past three decades, and the influence of Papanicolaou and Traut extends far beyond the cancer field.

In addition to the "Pap" test, other types of screening for noninfectious diseases evolved. Some of this was directed at the young. It was recognized that congenital dislocation of the hip could be detected in newborns by a simple physical examination (Ferrer, 1968). Schoolchildren were examined for heart defects (Association for the Prevention and Relief of Heart Disease, 1921). More generally, as acute infectious diseases were being brought under control, other conditions, especially vascular heart disease and cancers, were becoming increasingly important. With few exceptions, methods of preventing or treating these diseases were unsatisfactory, but it seemed logical that early intervention would be helpful. Although cancer, for instance, was often fatal, patients whose disease was treated while still localized were comparatively likely to survive (Greenough et al, 1924).

The American Society for the Control of Cancer (later the American Cancer Society) was organized in 1913; the Association for the Prevention and Relief of Heart Disease (later the American Heart Association) was formed in 1915. The goals of both organizations included early detection (Association for the Prevention and Relief of Heart Disease, 1921; Powers, 1921). In an analysis of the public health activities of this period, Winslow (1923) described the movement toward "the medical examination of well persons or of those in the early and incipient stages of disease. . . ." Winslow went on to write:

> Such programs involve a corresponding expansion of the application of medical services for the early diagnosis of disease, and call for a complete reconsideration of the function of the physician in modern community life. The control of the degenerative diseases requires nothing less than the systematic medical examination of presumably normal individuals, not merely of mothers and infants, of school children and tuberculous suspects, but of as large a section as possible of the entire population over forty-five years of age. It seems logically inevitable that such an application of medical knowledge shall, in some fashion, be provided, if medical science is to yield the high service of which it is capable, and which it can by no possibility render so long as it is limited to the alleviation of the symptoms of architecturally completed disease.

The Metropolitan Life Insurance Company (1921) suggested that annual physical examinations resulted in lower mortality rates. The idea that regular checkups are useful appears in Rosenau's *Preventive Medicine and Hygiene* beginning with the 1927 edition.

The search for asymptomatic conditions is now accepted as an important feature of medical care. Routine examinations and tests are aspects of "health promotion" (Commission on Chronic Illness, 1957; Wechsler et al, 1983), and comprehensive recommendations have been made for periodic examinations throughout life in order to detect and treat many diseases (Task Force, 1980). Winslow recognized, as have others more recently, that a serious effort to control diseases by early detection and treatment would lead to a basic change in the nature of medical practice.

No longer does it concern only a small number of ill persons, but large numbers of well persons are given advice as to when and how they should be examined for various diseases during their early, asymptomatic phases.

The set of procedures for early detection and treatment of a disease that is available to a population can be considered to be a *screening program.* A program can be divided into its diagnostic and therapeutic components. Both components are included in the term *screening program* because early detection must be followed by treatment to be useful in disease control. The diagnostic component includes the screening test(s), the screening schedule, and the procedures for diagnostic evaluation of people with positive tests. The therapeutic component is the process by which confirmed cases are treated. Obviously, there are many practical aspects of screening as well—the specific techniques used, the training of those who do the testing, the setting in which screening and, if necessary, treatment, is done, and so on.

Both the diagnostic and therapeutic components of a program have effects on a screened population. The diagnostic effects are those related to case detection and confirmation: the frequency of positive tests, the proportion confirmed and the amount of advancement in their times of diagnosis, and the frequency of false positives and the morbidity that these entail. The therapeutic effects, which determine the disease-control value of a screening program, are the postponement of serious morbidity or death, and any adverse effects of treatment that would not have existed were it not for the program. The therapeutic effects of a program depend, of course, on advancement in the time of diagnosis. Otherwise the diagnostic activities constitute a liability—they are expensive, and carry some risk. Therefore, a reduction in morbidity or mortality brought about by a screening program should outweigh the costs and adverse effects of early detection.

The success of a screening program at meeting this objective depends on interrelations between the disease experience of the target population, the characteristics of the screening procedures, and the effectiveness of the methods of treating disease early. The balance of this chapter summarizes these relationships and approaches to evaluating the diagnostic and therapeutic effects of screening programs. Formal definitions and detailed descriptions of methods are presented in later chapters.

CHARACTERISTICS OF DISEASE

To be suitable for control by a program of early detection and treatment, a disease must pass through a preclinical phase during which it is undiag-

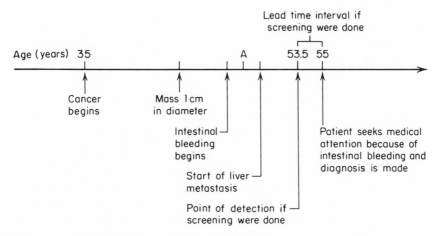

Figure 1–1. Preclinical phase of a hypothetical case of cancer of the colon.

nosed but detectable, and early treatment must offer some advantage over later treatment (Cole and Morrison, 1980). Obviously, there is no point in screening for a disease that cannot be detected before symptoms bring it to medical attention. And, if early treatment is not especially helpful, there is no point in early detection. The preclinical phase of a disease begins when the pathologic process is first present. For most if not all diseases, this point is ill defined. Signs that can be detected—such as a mass, exfoliating malignant cells, abnormal bleeding, or biochemical changes—develop later and more or less gradually. If no screening is done, the preclinical phase ends when the affected person seeks medical attention because symptoms have become apparent, and a diagnosis is made. Screening is usually directed at diseases that progress to an increasingly serious stage unless treated successfully. Even in a disease that is generally progressive, however, there may be some cases in which early disease does not progress but either disappears or remains asymptomatic indefinitely.

Figure 1–1 illustrates the preclinical phase of the natural history of a hypothetical case of cancer of the colon. The disease begins at age 35. Subsequently, a tumor mass develops, intestinal bleeding begins, and liver metastasis occurs, before the person recognizes any symptoms. The person seeks medical attention because of apparent intestinal bleeding, and a diagnosis is made, at age 55; this is the end of the preclinical phase. Figure 1–1 illustrates only one case, and as in any disease, there might be substantial case-to-case variation. Cases might progress slowly or rapidly, and specific manifestations might progress at different rates. In one case there might be no bleeding from the tumor during the preclinical phase, but symptoms from a large, very advanced, invading mass ultimately would lead to diagnosis. In another case, there might be substantial bleeding that would lead to diagnosis before the tumor mass has become large or has invaded very far. Because of such variation, a group of people with pre-clinical disease will include cases with a *distribution* of manifestations. Some will have no apparent signs; others will have manifestations that range from minimal to relatively advanced.

The point in its natural history at which a disease is typically diagnosed in a population depends on the availability of medical care and the level of medical awareness. Medical care already includes considerable screen-ing: Blood pressure, intraocular pressure, and urine sugar are often mea-sured on asymptomatic persons, and Pap smears are done extensively. The level of medical awareness determines the point in the development of a disease at which patients themselves tend to discover it. Ongoing screening and the level of medical awareness may be related: People are likely to be sensitive to their own symptoms in areas where screening is widespread. Therefore, the preclinical phase of a disease is taken to mean the period during which the disease remains undiagnosed in the *absence* of a *new* screening program under consideration. If prevailing medical conditions do not include any screening for the disease, then the preclinical phase corresponds to the period during which the disease is not perceived as symptomatic. Much of the discussion in this monograph takes this per-spective. If, on the other hand, some screening is already taking place, as with hypertension, then some cases of clinical disease will still be asymp-tomatic. Cases that are discovered by the new screening program are con-sidered to remain in the preclinical phase until they would have been dis-covered under prevailing conditions.

The proportion of a population that has detectable preclinical disease—its prevalence—is an important determinant of the utility of screening in controlling the disease. If the disease is extremely rare, screening will not be rewarding. The prevalence depends, first, on the incidence rate of the condition, which depends, in turn, on the action of causal factors. Second, the prevalence of preclinical disease varies with the average length of the preclinical phase. The longer the average duration, the higher the propor-tion of affected people. Third, the prevalence of undiagnosed but detect-able preclinical disease depends on whether or not the population has been screened previously. Recent screening of a population will have reduced the amount of undiagnosed disease and may change the pattern of signs of these cases. Suppose a population is screened for colon cancer with a test for occult blood in the stool. After screening, the proportion of people with undiagnosed preclinical colon cancer would be less than it was before screening, and the relative frequency of bleeding, compared to nonbleeding, tumors would be reduced.

The comparatively long duration of the preclinical phase of chronic compared to acute diseases is one reason that screening is directed almost exclusively at chronic conditions. It is usually feasible to detect and treat a high proportion of cases early only for diseases in which the preclinical phase is long. If the preclinical phase is short, virtually continuous re-screening would be necessary to meet that objective. Genetic diseases or congenital abnormalities such as phenylketonuria, Down syndrome, and neural tube defects are exceptions to the need for a long preclinical phase. The manifestations that are tested for are present at times that are known quite precisely in relation to conception or birth. Thus testing need only be done once.

Continued progression of a disease ultimately may lead to serious morbidity, such as symptomatic metastases or disability, and death. As indicated at the outset, the long-term goal of early detection and treatment is to reduce the frequency of these events. For this goal to be achieved, the expected rates of disability or death must be fairly high among the detected cases, early treatment must reduce these rates substantially, and the screen-detected cases must account for a substantial proportion of all disability or death from the disease.

CHARACTERISTICS OF SCREENING

The immediate purpose of screening is to designate people with preclinical disease as positive and people without preclinical disease as negative. The result of screening—a positive or negative designation—reflects both a test for signs of preclinical disease and a procedure for interpreting the findings. An error—a positive designation for someone without preclinical disease, or a negative designation for someone with it—can stem from either the test itself or its interpretation.

Examples of screening tests are an x-ray examination, a cytology examination, and a blood pressure determination. Obviously, incorrect measurements may be obtained. An x-ray film might fail, through poor technique, to reveal a mass that should be detectable; a mass present on x-ray might be overlooked; a mass might be "seen" on a film when one is not, in fact, present. A cytologic specimen might not have included malignant cells that were present, or the true degree of abnormality in a cytologic specimen might be under- or overstated. A person's blood pressure at the time of testing might be higher or lower than that person's typical blood pressure, or the reported blood pressure might differ from the actual value.

Even if there is no important error in a screening-test measurement, its interpretation—the assignment of a positive or negative outcome—may be incorrect. Often, if not always, the manifestation on which the test is based is found in some people without, as well as those with, the disease, and some people with preclinical disease might not have the manifestation. Masses visible on the mammogram occur in women without breast cancer; some women with breast cancer do not have masses on x-ray. Because of possible overlap of test measurements between diseased and well people, the interpretation of the test usually involves a *criterion of positivity*, the condition that must be met for a measurement to be considered positive. The criterion usually is a point on a scale extending from clearly normal to clearly abnormal. Errors of interpretation will reflect the location of the criterion. If the location is high (only very large masses on x-ray, or very malignant-appearing cells in a cytology specimen, are called positive), diseased people with only a moderate degree of abnormality on test will be designated negative (false negatives). Conversely, if the criterion of positivity is low (small or questionable masses on x-ray, or slightly atypical cells in a cytology specimen, are called positive, as are more severe changes), nondiseased people whose test results are even slightly abnormal will be labeled positive (false positives).

The ability of a test to designate people with preclinical disease as positive is referred to as the *sensitivity* of the test. A test will be called positive in a person with preclinical disease if a manifestation of the disease is detected and the degree of change exceeds the criterion of positivity. Customarily, sensitivity is defined as the proportion of cases with a positive screening test among all cases of preclinical disease, as identified by a positive diagnostic test. This definition poses certain problems. The most serious one is the frequent impossibility of applying a diagnostic test, which may be a surgical procedure, to asymptomatic people in order to determine who has the disease. Nonetheless, the concept of sensitivity is basic; a necessary feature of any screening program is a test that identifies the disease while it is in the preclinical phase. Moreover, it is important to be able to compare screening tests with respect to their abilities to detect early disease. The detected prevalence of preclinical disease is a useful and readily available indicator of the adequacy of sensitivity. Obviously, the more sensitive the test, the greater is the prevalence that will be detected in a given population, other things being equal. The sensitivities of different tests can be compared in terms of the prevalence of preclinical disease detected by each. Another measure of the sensitivity of a test is the number of cases detected during a screening program divided by the total number diagnosed, whether or not screen-detected.

The *specificity* of a test is its ability to designate as negative people who are not diseased. A test will be called negative in a nondiseased person provided that the test measurement obtained does not exceed the criterion of positivity. The specificity of a test determines whether or not the frequency of false positives will be low enough for a screening program to be feasible.

Sensitivity and specificity measure the ability of a test to identify correctly diseased and nondiseased people. In contrast, the *reliability* of a test is its capacity to give the same result—positive or negative, whether correct or incorrect—on repeated application in a person with a given level of disease. Reliability depends on the variability in the manifestation on which the test is based (eg, short-term fluctuation in blood pressure), and on the variability in the method of measurement and the skill with which it is made. The preliminary assessment of a screening test may include studies of its reliability. Although reliability does not guarantee high sensitivity and specificity, an unreliable test will probably not be sufficiently sensitive or specific to be useful. On the other hand, a test that is highly sensitive must be highly reliable when applied repeatedly to a diseased person, since a highly sensitive test would nearly always give the same result, that is, positive. Similarly, a test that is highly specific must be highly reliable when applied repeatedly to a well person.[1]

LEAD TIME: Visualize the course of preclinical disease in relation to screening in an individual case. At the onset of the disease and very early in its course, there are no detectable signs. In the case of colon cancer illustrated in Figure 1–1, there is initially no mass and no bleeding. The length of time during which no manifestation is detectable depends on the test used. However, it is always possible to envision some period during which there are no signs of the disease. As the disease develops, the manifestation that might be detected by the screening test begins to be present, but initially to only a small extent. For example, a very small mass is present or there is a small amount of bleeding. During this period, a screening test almost certainly would be negative since the manifestation is quite obscure. As the disease continues to progress, the manifestation becomes increasingly evident and if a test is done it is increasingly likely to be positive. After some time the manifestation reaches a state in which it probably would be detected if the test were done. If the disease remains undetected, continued progression leads to symptoms and the affected person seeks medical care. At this point the case is no longer eligible to be screened.

Suppose that a person with preclinical disease is screened and a positive test is obtained and confirmed by diagnostic tests. The interval from detection to the time at which diagnosis would have been made without that screening is known as the *lead time* (Figure 1–1) (Hutchison and Shapiro, 1968). The lead time depends on when screening is done in relation to the end of the preclinical phase. In Figure 1–1 the disease would be detected by screening 1.5 years before symptoms led to diagnosis. Just as the entire duration of preclinical disease might vary from person to person, the length of the lead-time interval might vary. In any group of cases detected in a screening program, some might have very short lead times. These are close to the development of symptoms; most of their preclinical phase has already passed when screening is done. Other cases might have intermediate or long lead times because the disease has been detected earlier in the preclinical phase. A person in whom nonprogressive preclinical disease is detected has an indefinitely long lead time, since that disease would never come to medical attention otherwise.

Lead time reflects the diagnostic pressure created by a screening program. The lead time created by screening is relative to the situation that would exist without it. Thus, a program aimed at increasing the level of breast self-examination might be of little value in a population that is frequently screened by mammography. The establishment of a screening program could also increase the earliness of routine diagnosis by increasing a population's awareness of symptoms (Chamberlain, 1982). This change could reduce the lead time, and subsequent health gains, brought about by the screening procedures themselves.

The idea of lead time is central to the rationale of disease control by early detection and treatment. Lead time is the amount of time by which treatment is "early." For a screening program to be effective in reducing morbidity or mortality in a population, there must be enough lead time in a sufficient number of cases. If lead time is insufficient, cases will not be treated in time to retard or stop their ultimate progression. If too few cases are detected, then early treatment, no matter how effective, will not have an important impact on the disease burden. The case in Figure 1–1 would not have been detected early enough for treatment to be very helpful since liver metastases had already occurred. On the other hand, detection at point A, before metastases were present, might have been curative.

The lead-time interval experienced by an individual person with screen-detected disease usually cannot be determined, since disease detected by screening is treated and there is no way to know when diagnosis would have occurred as a result of symptoms. However, the *distribution* of lead times created by a screening program can be evaluated by comparing the frequency of diagnosed cases, by time, between the screened group and a similar unscreened group (Morrison, 1982b). Thus, it is possible to estimate the proportions of screen-detected cases that have lead times that lie within specified limits (eg, less than one year, one to two years, three to four years, etc.). Estimation of the lead-time distribution is analogous to estimation of the beneficial effect of therapy for a disease such as cancer.

It is not possible to determine whether a given patient is cured by the treatment. However, it is possible to determine how many more treated than untreated patients survive for times that lie within specified limits. The distribution of lead times in a screening program depends on the sensitivity characteristics of the test, the frequency with which it is applied, and the incidence rate and distribution of the duration of preclinical disease. The detected prevalence of preclinical disease—one measure of test sensitivity—is a component of the lead-time distribution.

EFFECTIVENESS OF EARLY TREATMENT

Formal evaluation of early treatment is not always necessary. The detection and treatment of vision and hearing defects in children, for example, have benefits that are immediate and obvious. The only important issue for evaluation is the frequency with which such screening is done: Important defects should not go uncorrected for long, but screening should not be done so frequently as to be unnecessarily costly. For most diseases, however, the gains are not measurable until months or years have passed, and it is not possible to distinguish clearly the people who have, and have not, benefited from early treatment. As a result, careful study is usually required to ascertain the value of a screening program.

The primary determinants of the success of early treatment are the distribution of lead times generated by screening and the degree to which these lead times improve the effectiveness of treatment. In certain circumstances, early treatment can be evaluated separately from early detection. This is possible when there is uncertainty regarding the urgency of treatment of a screen-detected condition. For example, there was some question as to whether the advantages of treating mild hypertension outweigh the drawbacks (Fries, 1982). Therefore, the value of early treatment has been assessed by means of experiments comparing subsequent morbidity or mortality in treated v untreated screen-detected cases (Chapter 10).

In contrast to mild hypertension, there are many diseases in which treatment inevitably follows early diagnosis. It would be considered unthinkable not to treat screen-detected breast cancer. Moreover, an excision biopsy for diagnosis might be therapeutic. As a result, the diagnostic and therapeutic components of screening must be studied as a unit; it would not be possible to compare the course of treated v untreated screen-detected breast cancer. A study of early diagnosis and treatment combined is much more difficult to carry out than is a study of therapy alone, but a combined study is also the best way to assess the overall value of a given program of early detection, including the adverse effects owing to false positives.

Therefore, this book emphasizes the assessment of early treatment as part of the overall evaluation of a screening program.

Until recently there had been few properly designed studies of the value of screening programs, so that relatively little is known of the effectiveness of this form of disease control. Unfortunately, valid methods of evaluation were not widely understood until long after screening activities became firmly entrenched in medical practice, for two important reasons. First, there is a compelling intuitive appeal to the idea that earlier treatment *must* be better than later treatment. It seems inconceivable that there might be no gain in finding disease early. Second, some approaches to evaluation lead to erroneous results that tend to be unduly optimistic and reinforce the appeal of screening.

The most common method of attempting to evaluate the outcome of screening has been to compare the survival (or case fatality) of screen-detected cases with the survival of cases diagnosed because of the occurrence of symptoms. Survival is usually measured as the proportion of cases that survives a stated period after diagnosis, say, five years. Case fatality is one minus the survival, or the proportion of cases that die within a given time after diagnosis. The apparent implication of longer survival among screen-detected cases is that early treatment leads to prolonged life. However, a comparison of the survival of screen-detected *v* routinely diagnosed cases is impossible to interpret without additional information that usually is not available. There are two diagnostic effects of screening that may result in a higher survival in screen-detected cases than in routinely diagnosed cases, and these factors are not separated readily from the therapeutic effect of early treatment. First, patients whose disease is detected by screening gain lead time—the diagnosis of their disease is earlier than the time that clinical diagnosis would have occurred. Even if the time of death is unchanged, the proportion of cases that survive for some period after diagnosis (and the proportion of low-stage cases) will increase as a result of earlier diagnosis alone. Second, screening may tend to identify cases destined to have a relatively benign course even if there is no lead time or reduction in mortality from early treatment. Such *prognostic selection* would occur if screening preferentially detects disease with a long preclinical phase *(length-biased sampling)*. Presumably, patients with such disease also would have a long clinical phase, that is, favorable survival. In short, comparisons of case fatality or survival are likely to suggest a benefit even if none exists, and may greatly exaggerate the size of a true benefit as it would be reflected in the mortality rate of a screened population.

In the last two decades there has been an increased awareness of the special problems of evaluating early diagnosis and treatment. A study of screening for breast cancer, undertaken by researchers at the Health

Insurance Plan of Greater New York (HIP) (Shapiro et al, 1988), has been the predominant stimulus to the development of epidemiologic methods in this area. The ultimate gains derived from a screening program are reductions of serious illness and death among the people screened. For a study to be valid, the observed relation between the program and the rate of morbidity or mortality should reflect only the amount of gain derived from the program and not other differences between screened and unscreened groups. For example, screening leads to diagnosis of disease earlier than it would occur otherwise, so that a screened population will have a higher rate of diagnosis than will an unscreened population that is similar in other respects. Therefore, the evaluation of screening must be based on measures of disease occurrence that will not be affected by early diagnosis except to the extent that early treatment is beneficial.

One such measure is the overall mortality rate—the rate of death from all causes. Other things being equal, the mortality rate will be lower in a screened than an unscreened group only if early treatment prevents or postpones death from the disease screened for. However, the change in the overall mortality rate has an important drawback as a measure of efficacy. Frequently, the target disease accounts for only a small fraction of all deaths in a population. If this is the case, the overall mortality rate will be quite insensitive to a beneficial effect of screening. For example, even a marked reduction in breast cancer mortality would have only a small effect on the rate of mortality from all causes; a beneficial effect of screening for breast cancer might not be demonstrable by means of overall mortality rates.

The disease-specific mortality rate (eg, the breast cancer mortality rate) is a much more sensitive measure, and, in many circumstances, it will be the primary outcome to be assessed. Like the overall mortality rate, the *true* underlying disease-specific rate will not be changed by early diagnosis alone. It is possible, however, that the time and manner of initial diagnosis do affect cause-of-death certification, and, therefore, the *measured* rate. A more serious problem is that the appropriate rates for study can be difficult to identify. The entities that might be favorably affected by early treatment may not be certain. In screening to control cardiovascular disease, for example, the intervention may affect heart attack, stroke, sudden death, and possibly other categories. Furthermore, the value of a screening program is reduced by its adverse effects, those of early treatment and those suffered by false-positive screenees. Disease-specific mortality rates selected for attention should also reflect the adverse effects of screening.

Because screening leads to early diagnosis, the relation of screening to morbidity is quite difficult to assess. A means must be devised to separate actual morbidity caused by the disease or its treatment from apparent morbidity that is the result only of the designation of persons as diseased because of screening. One way to accomplish this goal is to establish operational definitions of morbidity based on disease that is severe enough to ensure diagnosis even without screening. For example, a woman might be considered to become ill from breast cancer when she first develops symptoms from metastases of the disease. A diagnosis of breast cancer, without symptoms of spread, would not be considered as breast cancer morbidity. Thus, the morbidity rate from breast cancer would be taken as the incidence rate of symptomatic metastases. If a screened population had a lower rate than an unscreened population, this finding would be evidence that screening and early treatment protect against the development of late-stage cancer. Similarly, in a study of screening for hypertension, the rate of development of symptomatic myocardial infarction might be taken as a measure of morbidity; asymptomatic electrocardiographic changes would not be taken into account.

METHODS: Evaluation of the efficacy of screening can be accomplished by means of either experimental or nonexperimental methods. The experimental approach involves comparisons of mortality (or morbidity) between groups that have and have not been assigned to the program being evaluated. The groups are best constituted by randomization. Experimental evaluation is exemplified by the HIP trial. About 31,000 women (the study group) were offered an initial screening examination (mammography and physical examination) for breast cancer followed by three additional examinations at yearly intervals; about 20,000 women had one or more of the examinations. Another 31,000 women (the control group), similar to the study group in age and other characteristics, were not offered the screening program but were selected by the same procedure as was the group offered the program. After ten years the cumulative mortality from breast cancer was about 30% lower in the study group than in the control group. These results indicate the efficacy of the program of early diagnosis and treatment in reducing breast cancer mortality.

The advantages of experimental studies are well known. The most important is that potential confounding factors—determinants of morbidity or mortality other than the program being evaluated—will, on the average, be distributed equally between the screened and control groups as a result of the random allocation of subjects. Moreover, these determinants will tend to be evenly distributed even if they are difficult to measure or unknown. Therefore, a properly conducted experimental study provides a valid estimate of the gains that can be achieved by screening. With the data from such a study, it is also possible to analyze the effects that early treatment, lead time, and prognostic selection have on the survival of patients with screen-detected disease (Morrison, 1982b).

There are, however, serious obstacles to conducting experimental studies of screening. Many thousands of subjects may have to be enrolled and kept under observation for years. Because of the logistical problems and expense involved, large studies can be used to answer only the most urgent questions. Because of the time involved, experimental assessment may not be able to keep pace with changes in screening technology. Finally, it may not be acceptable to either physicians or potential study subjects to participate in an experimental study of a procedure such as the Pap smear that is established in medical practice. Owing to these difficulties there is a role for nonexperimental evaluation of the effectiveness of early diagnosis and treatment.

There are three basic nonexperimental approaches: follow-up or cohort studies, case-control studies, and correlation (ecologic) studies. A follow-up study involves the determination and comparison of advanced illness or death rates between people who choose to be screened at a given time and those who do not. A case-control study involves the determination of screening history in people who have developed advanced disease or die from it and in a comparison group of unaffected people. This information can be used to relate the rate of development of advanced disease, or death, to screening history. A correlation study describes the relation between the screening patterns and the disease experiences of several populations.

Nonexperimental studies are more likely than experimental studies to suffer from confounding. For example, screening experience depends on personal choices that may be related to subsequent morbidity or mortality through "health awareness." However, confounding by health awareness might not be suspected and, therefore, not controlled. The effects of even known confounding factors may not be completely controllable. Suppose that income were used to adjust for social class in a study of screening for cervical cancer. Income might not embody all the relevant aspects of social class, leading to residual confounding. On the other hand, income might be the appropriate factor to control, but subjects might err in reporting it, again resulting in residual confounding (Greenland, 1980).

Even if confounding factors were completely controlled, the implications of a nonexperimental study for screening policy may not be clear. Correlation studies are often concerned with average screening frequencies in populations, not the frequencies with which individuals are screened. Follow-up and case-control studies are likely to require special attention to design and analysis in order to avoid bias in relating screening, and especially screening frequency, to mortality or advanced morbidity.

Finally, the quality of the data collected may not be as good in nonexperimental studies as in experiments. Typically, nonexperimental studies must rely on information assembled for other purposes or on the memories of subjects. Random errors in the information (errors in data on screening experience that do not depend on outcome, or errors in data on outcome that do not depend on screening experience) would tend to obscure the effects of screening. Of even more concern are errors in assessing exposure status that are related to outcome. It might be difficult to distinguish true screening examinations from tests done to investigate symptomatic illness. If so, the value of screening would be underestimated. People who have developed metastases from a cancer might be overly likely to report that they had not been screened. This type of error would lead to an overestimate of the protective effect of screening.

To summarize, experimental evaluation of screening is seriously hindered by the size of these studies, their length, and the attendant cost. Nonexperimental methods may be of some help, but cannot be depended on to provide all the information that may be required.

FEASIBILITY OF SCREENING

To be suitable for general use, a program of early detection and treatment should meet several criteria in addition to reducing morbidity or mortality. The screening procedures must be convenient and virtually free of discomfort or risk. Screening must be attractive to members of the target population; the people must be screened efficiently and economically; positive screenees must have appropriate diagnostic studies; and confirmed cases must be treated. In addition to these administrative features, the program should lead to a high level of case detection and a reasonably low level of false-positive test results.

The level of case detection depends on the prevalence of preclinical disease in the population screened and on the sensitivity characteristics of the test used. If the frequency of detection is too low, the cost per case will be too high. Furthermore, the reduction of morbidity or mortality will be small. Although the prevalence of preclinical disease is related to both its incidence and its duration, the duration is the more important determinant of the feasibility of screening and early treatment as a method of disease control. For a given prevalence, the proportion of cases in the preclinical state, and the ones potentially benefited by a screening program, rises as the average duration rises (and the incidence rate falls).

The frequency of false positives depends almost entirely on the specificity of the test used. The consequences of false positives are flooding of diagnostic services, possible adverse effects of the diagnostic tests that must be done, and high costs.

The sensitivity or specificity of screening may be enhanced by technical improvements in the test used. Either sensitivity or specificity also may be increased, but at the expense of the other, by the use of multiple tests in various sequences or by adjustment of the criterion of positivity. Often, however, very high sensitivity can be obtained only if the specificity is unacceptably low.

The *predictive value* (PV) in a screening program is the proportion of people with a positive test, who are found by diagnostic evaluation to have the disease in question (Vecchio, 1966). A high PV suggests that a reasonably high proportion of the costs of a program are in fact being expended for the detection of disease during its preclinical phase. A low PV suggests that a high proportion of the costs are being wasted on the detection and diagnostic evaluation of false positives, people who have positive screening tests but not the disease. It is important to emphasize, however, that the PV is a proportional measure; a high PV might be obtained even if the frequency of case detection is low and the corresponding reduction in mortality is small.

The determinants of the PV of a given screening examination are the specificity and sensitivity of the test and the prevalence of preclinical disease in the target population. A low PV is more likely to be the result of poor specificity than of poor sensitivity. It is the specificity that determines the number of false positives. False positives are derived from people without the disease, who constitute the vast majority of people tested in virtually any program. Although the *proportion* of false positives might be small, even a small loss of specificity can lead to a large increase in their *number,* and a large decline in the PV. An increase in sensitivity will increase the number of true positives and, therefore, the PV. However, care must be taken to achieve any increase in sensitivity with little or no loss of specificity. For a test with a given sensitivity and specificity, the PV increases with the prevalence. Therefore, the PV of a screening program can be improved by restricting the program to people at high risk, that is, those who have a relatively high prevalence of preclinical disease, or by screening at a lower frequency to maintain the prevalence of preclinical disease in the target population at a higher level. Either approach leads to some overall loss of the value of screening since fewer cases are detected and treated early.

It should be apparent from the foregoing discussion that it is not enough simply to know that early treatment can reduce morbidity or mortality from a disease. The effect of screening may be too small to be valuable, or a program of disease control based on screening may be impossibly expensive or impractical for other reasons. Therefore, the long-term goal of studying the early diagnosis and treatment of a disease is formulation of a realistic screening policy—a specification of who should be screened, at what ages, and with what tests—in order to put practical and rewarding programs into operation. The availability of screening tests, and interest in using them, has far outstripped our knowledge of their characteristics and value. As a result, some present-day screening recommendations and activities are not well grounded. Screening policy should be based on a thorough understanding of the effects of early detection and treatment.

NOTE

[1]Figure 7–1 shows the dependence of sensitivity and specificity on reliability. Imagine a test that gives the same measurement on average but is less reliable than the one that led to the distributions shown. The resulting distributions would be centered around the same values, but they would be broader, so that a higher proportion of nonglaucomatous eyes would have intraocular pressures above 25 mm—reduced specificity—and a higher proportion of glaucomatous eyes would have pressures below 25 mm—reduced sensitivity.

2 The Natural History of Disease in Relation to Measures of Disease Frequency

Nearly all important issues in screening—the capabilities of tests, the efficacy of early treatment, the utility of a screening program in a given population, and methods of evaluating these characteristics—are linked to the natural history of the target disease: the rate at which it progresses, the signs and symptoms that it causes, and changes in its susceptibility to therapy. Many aspects of natural history that are influenced by screening cannot be observed directly in individual cases but are reflected in measures of disease frequency. Therefore, an understanding of screening includes the ability to interpret changes in disease frequency in a screened population with respect to changes in individual cases. This chapter describes the components of the natural history, their relationship to basic measures of disease frequency, and the changes in these measures as related to changes in natural history brought about by early detection and treatment.

Cancer of the cervix provides one of the best examples of the natural history of a disease suitable for screening. An accepted concept of the progressive development of this disease, from dysplasia to invasive cancer, is shown in Figure 2–1. The preinvasive phases—dysplasia and carcinoma in situ—typically evolve over years or decades, allowing ample time for detection. These periods, however, might be highly variable. There might be instances in which the phase of carcinoma in situ is nonexistent, or at least very short. If so, there would be cases of invasive cancer that could not have been detected while in the in situ phase. On the other hand, there might be cases of dysplasia or carcinoma in situ that do not progress further, or that even regress to earlier phases (Boyes et al, 1982; Task Force, 1976).

A general illustration of the natural history of a case of a disease for which screening might be considered is given in Figure 2–2a. This diagram was developed from a scheme given by Hutchison (1960). Each point represents the age of the case at the time of the indicated event. The biologic onset of the disease occurs at point A, the start of the preclinical phase. This point may be poorly defined or not observable. In cancer, for example, this could be the point at which a transformed cell is first present. Point A′ is the point at which the disease is first detectable by the screening test to be used. For example, point A′ might refer to the time at which a cancer mass reaches the minimum size that can be seen on an x-ray. Obviously, the location of point A′, and the probability that a case could be detected at it, depends on the screening technique.

As a result of progression of the disease, symptoms appear that bring the patient to medical attention and treatment at point B. This is the end of the preclinical phase, which is the period of time from A to B. Point B also marks the start of the clinical phase of the natural history. Continued progression of the disease would lead to severe or disabling illness—such as symptomatic metastases of cancer—at point C, and the patient dies from the disease at point D. Thus, the clinical phase is the period from B to D. Obviously, the times from initial symptoms to advanced illness or death may reflect the effects of treatments given, as well as the underlying characteristics of the untreated disease. "Death from the disease" means a death that occurs when it does because the disease of interest is present. Most such deaths would be certified as due to the disease, but some may not. A death that occurs when it does because a cancer is present, but with the cause of death certified as pneumonia or heart failure is, in principal, a cancer death, although it might not be counted that way in a study.

Figure 2–2 suggests that point B, the time of diagnosis and treatment, would immediately follow the occurrence of symptoms. Perceptible symptoms in a person not yet known to have the disease might be classified at one of three levels. At the most severe level are symptoms that lead such a person to seek medical attention, regardless of whether screening is available. These symptoms signal the end of the preclinical phase in usual circumstances. An intermediate level of symptoms probably exists that would bring a person to a newly established (and publicized) screening program but not to routine sources of medical care. Therefore, a new program

Figure 2–1. Natural history of the preclinical phase of carcinoma of the cervix.

Source: Based on Task Force (1976).

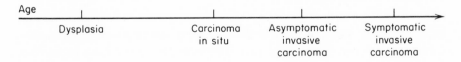

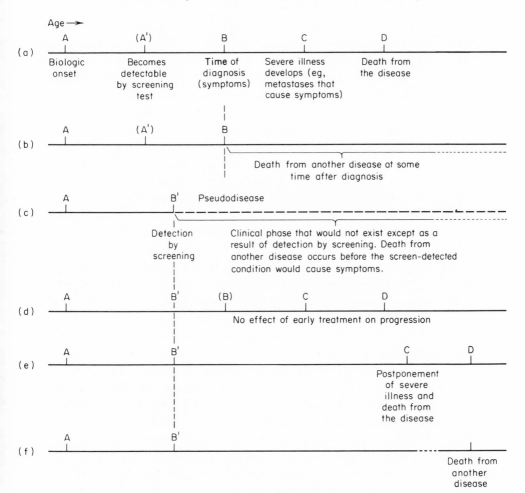

Figure 2–2. Illustration of some aspects of the natural history of disease.

might appear more successful at casefinding than it would be later on. The minimum level consists of perceptible symptoms that can be elicited by questioning but that do not lead the affected person to take any action. Operationally, diagnosis, rather than symptoms, signals the end of the preclinical phase. The time from consulting a physician to establishing a diagnosis is nearly always very short relative to the length of either the preclinical or the clinical phase. Therefore, in the absence of any screening it is appropriate to assume that symptomatic cases are clinical, recognizing that there may be undiagnosed cases with intermediate or minimal symptoms.

The presence of disease at a certain level might lead to the perception of a symptom by one person but not another, so that the time of diagnosis will vary from case to case, even among cases with the same age at biologic onset and the same growth characteristics. Other temporal aspects of disease illustrated in Figure 2–2 may also vary. The onset of the disease, and the beginning of detectability, might occur at different ages. The period of detectability might be short or long, and the ages at which advanced illness or death occur might differ.

Other types of natural histories can be envisioned. Fortunately, patients do not always die of their diseases, even serious ones like cancer. In such a case, the disease might never reappear after treatment; the person ultimately dies of an unrelated disease (Figure 2–2b). It is also possible to define *pseudodisease*, a lesion that becomes known only as a result of screening; it would not be discovered otherwise (Figure 2–2c). Conceptually, two types of pseudodisease can be distinguished: cases that would never progress to a symptomatic state (ie, those that regress from asymptomatic to normal or remain in the asymptomatic state indefinitely) and cases that would progress but are interrupted by death from unrelated diseases before symptoms develop. In principle, screening will always lead to the detection of some of the latter type of pseudodisease, but this would be unimportant unless the lead times of progressive cases are very long.

The amount of pseudodisease created by screening depends on the detected prevalence of preclinical disease and the rate at which the cases progress to symptomatic illness. The amount of pseudodisease provides a quantitative distinction between screening for a disease v screening for a risk factor. Most screen-detected cases of breast cancer (a disease) ultimately would become symptomatic. In contrast, only a minority of persons with screen-detected hypertension or hypercholesterolemia (risk factors) may develop stroke or myocardial infarction, depending on the criterion of positivity of the test.

Like any theoretical construct, a scheme of the natural history of a disease has some arbitrary features. For example, myocardial infarction and stroke, which are symptomatic manifestations of arteriosclerotic vascular disease, have several different predisposing conditions, such as hypertension, diabetes, and hyperlipidemia. If the focus of a screening program is the detection and treatment of hypertension, then it may be described as the preclinical disease, without reference to other precursors. Different schemes would be appropriate in screening for diabetes or hyperlipidemia. In screening to reduce deaths from cancer of the colon, the preclinical diseases of interest include benign adenomatous polyps, noninvasive cancer, and early stage invasive cancer. The relative proportions of the different lesions detected (and their anatomic distribution) will depend in part on whether screening is done by sigmoidoscopy or by testing for blood in the stool. Obviously, the length of the preclinical phase, and therefore the amount of time that must elapse before any benefit can result from early treatment, also depends on the type of early disease under consideration. If colonic adenomas are viewed as a precursor of colon cancer, the duration of the preclinical phase might be much longer than it would if this phase were limited to early cancer. If so, the value of detecting and removing colonic adenomas would take much longer to become evident than would the value of early treatment of cancer itself.

Concepts of the natural history of a disease frequently link components derived by different investigators in different ways. Observations on the clinical phase are usually made separately from observations on the preclinical phase. Events during the preclinical phase often must be inferred rather than observed directly. Thus, the progressively later average ages at diagnosis of cervical dysplasia, carcinoma in situ, microinvasive carcinoma, and symptomatic invasive cancer of the cervix in groups of patients are taken as support for the sequence of events shown for individuals in Figure 2–1. Some more direct evidence has been furnished by cytologic follow-up studies of patients with dysplasia or carcinoma in situ (Boyes et al, 1982; Task Force, 1976). The premalignant nature of dysplasia and carcinoma in situ of the cervix is most convincingly established by the demonstration that detecting and removing them leads to a reduction in mortality from cervical cancer (Chapter 11).

Screening is usually considered for diseases such as cancer, heart disease, and diabetes. These diseases are characterized by clinical courses that are chronic and progressive, but highly variable. In particular, there are no obvious criteria for when a cure of an individual case has been achieved. The disease might recur many years after apparently successful treatment in some cases but not in other similar cases. Therefore, certain useful conventions have evolved for describing the occurrence and natural history of serious chronic diseases. Once a diagnosis is made, the affected person is considered to be a "case" for the rest of his life. If the disease progresses (eg, if metastases develop), the person is from then on considered to have the later stage even if evidence of it is obliterated by treatment. Thus, an *individual* patient is never declared "cured." A *group* of patients is considered "cured" if the subsequent mortality of the group is the same as that of a comparable group without the disease (Cutler et al, 1969; Ederer et al, 1961).

INCIDENCE AND MORTALITY RATES

The frequency of diagnosis of a disease in a group of people is described by the corresponding incidence or morbidity rate. The frequency of death from this disease is described by the disease-specific mortality rate.

The *incidence rate* is the ratio of the number of newly diagnosed cases of that disease that occur in a group to the amount of person-time, usually expressed as person-years (PY), experienced by its members while under observation. Members of the group may enter it at different times. Each member contributes person-time to the denominator of the morbidity rate until the disease is diagnosed or until observation ends for some other reason such as death from another disease, or migration, or the end of the study. The incidence rate for a calendar period is the ratio of the number of cases that occur in the period to the person-time experienced during the same period.

The *mortality rate* relates the number of deaths from a disease to person-time. This includes person-time experienced by people known to have the disease of interest, as well as by clinically unaffected people. In contrast, the denominator of the incidence rate includes only person-time experienced by people who have not yet had the disease diagnosed. The computation and interpretation of incidence and mortality rates are described by Breslow and Day (1980, 42–49), Elandt-Johnson (1975), Morgenstern et al (1980), and Rothman (1986, 23–29).

It is crucial to distinguish the mortality rate in a population, some of whose members have the disease but most do not, from the mortality rate among cases, or the *case-fatality rate*. The preceding paragraph concerns the mortality rate in a population. This is the mortality rate that is often the focus of studies of disease causation, and this rate is one of the most useful measures of the value of screening programs. The case-fatality rate (CFR) is discussed at length in chapter 6. The CFR relates the number of deaths from a disease to person-time experienced only after diagnosis. The mortality rate from a disease in a population depends on the incidence rate and the CFR. The usual measures of the natural history of the clinical phase of a disease—survival or cumulative case fatality—are simple mathematical functions of the CFR.[1]

In a group of given size, the incidence rate of a disease depends on the number of cases that have begun to develop before the end of observation and on the distribution of the length of the preclinical phase. Only cases that complete the preclinical phase and are diagnosed during the observation period contribute to the numerator of the rate. The mortality rate depends on the number of cases diagnosed before the end of observation and the distribution of the length of the clinical phase. Only cases that complete the clinical phase (ie, die) during the observation period contribute to the numerator. A case does not contribute to the numerator of the *disease-specific* mortality rate for any period if the individual dies of a disease other than the one being studied. However, such a case would contribute person-time to the denominator up to the time of death.

Among people of a given age, the rates of initial diagnosis, advanced illness, and death from a disease are not affected by rates of removal from observation for other causes, provided that the risks are independent (Cornfield, 1957).

Rates based on disease events other than initial diagnosis and death can be defined. For example, the *advanced illness rate* is the number of cases of an advanced condition, such as symptomatic cancer metastases, that develop in relation to person-time in clinically well people and those with the diagnosed disease that has not yet progressed so far.

Even if all cases of a disease progress, the rate of each event shown in Figure 2–2a is less than the rate of the preceding events. That is, the mortality rate is less than the rate of development of advanced illness, which is, in turn, less than the rate of initial diagnosis. The reason for these differences is that the rate of each event is based on more person-time than are the rates of earlier events in the sequence (Morrison, 1979a). The incidence rate is based only on person-time experienced up to initial diagnosis; the rate of development of advanced illness is based on person-time experienced by clinically unaffected people *and* those with clinical disease that is not advanced, and the mortality rate is based on person-time without regard to disease state. These differences in rate would be small for a disease that progresses rapidly since the short time taken up by later phases of the natural history have little effect on the denominator. On the other hand, the differences would be large if the disease progresses slowly or if a substantial fraction of cases that reach a given stage do not progress further.

Incidence and mortality rates for most diseases vary with age. Therefore, measurements often are made on an age-specific basis. An age-specific rate is limited to events and person-time in a given age interval. A crude observed incidence or mortality rate for a disease depends on the age-specific rates and the age structure of the group observed. Suppose that rates rise with age, as is the case for many chronic diseases. Then, a group that has a high proportion of old people will have a higher crude rate than will an otherwise similar group with a low proportion of old people. For a group whose composition is fixed at the start of a period of observation— such as a group of subjects in an experimental trial—the age structure during the period will depend on the age-specific death rates from all causes and on the age-specific rates of loss to follow-up (or out-migration). If the composition of a group is not fixed, as would be the case for the population of a town, the age structure also will depend on rates of birth and immigration. To compare morbidity and mortality rates among groups with different age structures, age-specific rates can be adjusted by use of a standard age distribution (Rothman, 1986, 41–49).

CUMULATIVE INCIDENCE AND MORTALITY

In a group that is followed for a period of time, the proportion in whom a disease is diagnosed is defined as the *cumulative incidence* and the proportion that dies is defined as the *cumulative mortality*. These quantities depend on the incidence rate and mortality rate, respectively. The observed cumulative incidence and cumulative mortality from a given disease also depend on mortality from other causes. The higher the mortality from other causes, the lower are the observed cumulative incidence and mortality from the specified disease. However, it is possible to estimate what these quantities would be if there were no deaths from other causes (Chiang, 1961; Elandt-Johnson, 1975; Morgenstern et al, 1980; Rothman, 1986, 29–32). The *conditional* cumulative mortality is the estimated proportion dying from the disease in a period of time given that subjects are not removed from observation for reasons other than death from the disease of interest. The conditional cumulative incidence is the proportion diagnosed during the period, assuming no removal from observation for other reasons.[2]

The *unconditional* cumulative mortality is defined as the proportion of individuals that dies from the disease in the presence of other reasons for removal from observation, in particular, death from other diseases. It is equivalent to the observed cumulative mortality. The unconditional cumulative mortality for a specified set of circumstances may be estimated from the mortality rates from the disease of interest and from all causes.[3] The unconditional cumulative mortality is lower than the conditional cumulative mortality by an amount that depends on the mortality from all causes.

PREVALENCE

The prevalence of a condition is the proportion of a group affected at a particular time (or age). Under usual conditions (no new screening), the prevalence of clinical disease is the number of people with diagnosed disease divided by the total number of people in the group. The prevalence of preclinical disease relates the number diseased but not diagnosed to the total number of people exclusive of those with clinical disease. The latter are excluded because they cannot, by definition, have preclinical disease at the time specified.

The prevalence of preclinical disease at a given point depends on the number of cases in which the disease began earlier, and on the number of these in which the duration of the preclinical phase is long enough to encompass the specified point. Prevalent preclinical cases at that time would not include cases that began very early and had progressed to the clinical phase or cases that began relatively recently but had only brief preclinical phases. Thus, the prevalence tends to be high if the rate of disease initiation is high or if the length of the preclinical phase tends to be long. Similarly, the prevalence of clinical disease tends to be high if the diagnosis rate is high or if the length of the clinical phase tends to be long (Freeman and Hutchison, 1980). Extending the clinical phase after diagnosis (eg, by better treatment) leads to a higher prevalence of clinical disease but a lower mortality rate. In a group of people initially free of clinical disease and observed for a given period, the prevalent number of cases of clinical disease at the end of the period is equal to the cumulative number that become diagnosed minus the number of those people that die. The corresponding denominator is the total number of people at the start minus the cumulative number of deaths from all causes.

MORTALITY IN PERSONS ELIGIBLE TO BE SCREENED

A disease-specific mortality rate in the general population is based on deaths regardless of the time of diagnosis. Known cases of the disease, however, are not eligible to be screened. These cases otherwise would contribute to the observed mortality. Thus, mortality tends to be lower among persons eligible to be screened than it is in the general population. The difference will be especially large during the early years of a screening program. This difference should be taken into account in deriving the expected mortality to be compared to that observed in a screened group, and in planning the size of a study to evaluate screening.

The mortality among persons eligible to be screened (but who are not screened) depends on the incidence of the disease and its case fatality (Morrison, 1979a; Morrison et al, 1988; Morrison, 1991b). To estimate expected mortality, the expected incidence is determined according to time after the start of eligibility for screening (entry). Then, case fatality according to time since diagnosis is applied to the time-specific incidences. The total disease-specific mortality expected for a given period after entry is derived by summing the expected values for which the time intervals from entry to diagnosis, plus diagnosis to death, are equal.

For a given age at entry, the expected disease-specific cumulative mortalities, for individual years after entry, may be calculated as follows. The subscripts refer to time, which is defined as zero at entry. Years are indexed by the time at the end of the completed year.

Let

I_i = incidence rate of disease during year i after entry

S_1 = expected proportion of study participants that escape the risk of diagnosis of the disease through year $a-1$

$$S_1 = \exp\left(-\sum_{i=1}^{a-1} I_i\right)$$

c_a = expected proportion of persons diagnosed during year a

= $1 - \exp(-I_a)$

f_j = conditional cumulative case fatality (conditional cumulative mortality) from the disease among cases during year j after diagnosis

f_{T-a+1} = conditional cumulative case fatality from the disease during year T after entry, among cases diagnosed during year a after entry

S_2 = expected proportion of cases diagnosed during year a that survive the risk of death from the disease through year T-1

$$S_2 = \prod_{j=1}^{T-a} (1 - f_j)$$

Then,

M_T = expected cumulative mortality from the disease in year T after entry among persons eligible to be screened

$$M_T = \frac{\displaystyle\sum_{a=1}^{T} f_{T-a+1} S_2 C_a S_1}{\displaystyle\sum_{i=1}^{T-1} (1 - M_i)} \tag{2-1}$$

The components of this formula are $S_2 C_a S_1$, the proportion of cases that live up to, but not including, year T after entry, and f_{T-a+1}, the proportion of cases alive at the start of year T that die of the disease during year T. Thus, M_T can be viewed as the expected proportion of deaths during year T among extant cases, divided by the expected proportion of persons who survive the risk of death from the disease up to the start of year T. If the incidence of and mortality from the disease are low, M_T will be nearly equal to the expected mortality rate for the disease (deaths/PY) during year T.

Expression (2–1) is a central relationship in screening. The equation connects mortality to times of diagnosis and subsequent case fatality. The distribution of the lead time of screening is given by the differences in times of diagnosis between screened and unscreened persons. If the incidence and case-fatality data are derived from the screened population, expression (2–1) corresponds to the observed mortality in that group whether or not screening was beneficial (Table 8–2). The time-specific case fatalities are reduced in the screened group compared to the unscreened group by amounts that correspond to the distribution of lead time. If early treatment is effective, the case fatality in the screened group is reduced further.

With incidence and case fatality data from the source (or comparison) population, expression (2–1) gives the expected disease-specific mortality in the absence of a favorable effect of early treatment. The use of the expected mortality in a nonexperimental follow-up study is illustrated in chapter 5. The use of the expected mortality in planning the size of a study is illustrated in chapter 4. Expression (2–1) also can be expanded to allow prediction of the effect of early treatment based on the times of diagnosis and prognostic features of the cases (chapter 8).

EFFECTS OF SCREENING

Any case of disease that first comes to medical attention as the result of screening (that is not part of prevailing care) is, by definition, discovered during its preclinical phase. The amount of time by which the diagnosis is early is the lead time. In Figure 2–2d, the lead time is the interval from B′ to (B), the time that diagnosis would have occurred if screening had not been done. If a screening program is of any value, that value must be a consequence of advancement in the time of treatment of screen-detected cases. The amount of lead time necessary to favorably alter the natural history will vary from disease to disease and from case to case, and will depend on the treatment.

If early treatment has no effect on the progression of the disease, the ages at which advanced illness or death would ultimately occur are unchanged despite the lead time gained (Figure 2–2d). On the other hand, if early treatment is valuable, then advanced illness or death from the disease will either be postponed (Figure 2–2e) or will not occur at all (Figure 2–2f). This benefit must be experienced after point B, the time at which diagnosis would have occurred without screening. People in whom death from the disease is prevented, rather than simply postponed, have a normal life expectancy for their age. These people die of an unrelated cause, as if they had not had the screen-detected disease.

As mentioned previously, there might be some cases of asymptomatic disease—pseudodisease—that would never come to medical attention as a result of symptoms. Cases of pseudodisease that are detected by screening can not benefit from early treatment since they would not have had the disease clinically if they had not been screened (Figure 2–2c).

Hutchison (1960) postulated that there is a "critical point" in the evolution of each case of a disease. Treatment would be much more effective before this critical point than after. Therefore, a case that can only be cured by early treatment must have a lead time at least as long as the interval from the critical point to the time at which symptoms would have developed. Zelen (1976) applied this concept to population screening for breast cancer. If the critical point is the formation of metastases, then one can imagine a function that relates the average stage in the natural history at which cases are treated to the years of life a population loses because of the disease. The smaller the proportion of metastatic cases, whether as a result of screening or other characteristics of the population, the lower the mortality (Figure 2–3).

It may be more appropriate to think of a "critical interval" than a "critical point." The decline of curability probably does not occur instantly. In cancer, for example, the likelihood of cure might decrease as a function of the volume of metastatic tumor.

The location of the critical interval in the natural history is likely to vary from disease to disease, and from case to case for a given disease. In some cases of cancer, metastases may occur months or even years before the development of symptoms. Other cases probably are cured by treatment given after the occurrence of symptoms. The proportion of such cases is quite different for breast cancer than it is for lung cancer or pancreatic cancer. In coronary artery disease, there is a critical zone related to the occurence of extensive damage to heart muscle or to the electrical system of the heart. This transition may occur at about the time of initial symptoms (myocardial infarction or sudden death), or long after initial symptoms (angina pectoris).

There might be a complex relation of curability to time as the disease progresses. In coronary artery disease, for example, the chance of preventing a myocardial infarction would decrease when an arteriosclerotic plaque changes from simple to complex, thus increasing the probability of thrombosis (Wissler, 1985). There would be a second reduction in curability once a myocardial infarction actually occurs.

In order to relate changes in the natural history of an individual case to the corresponding changes in incidence and mortality rates, and the prevalence of preclinical and clinical disease, it is necessary to describe the schedule of screening. The schedule can be specified with respect to individual participants or an entire screened group. For an individual, the period of testing with a single screening examination is virtually instantaneous. For a group, however, the period of testing depends on the inten-

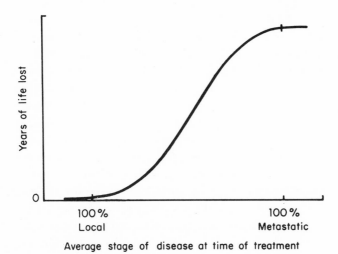

Figure 2–3. Hypothetical relation between average stage of disease at time of treatment in a population and years of life lost.

Source: Adapted from Zelen M: Theory of early detection of breast cancer in the general population. In Heuson JC, Mattheiem WH, Rozencweig M (eds). *Breast Cancer: Trends in Research and Treatment.* New York, Raven Press, 1976, Figure 3.

sity of screening activities: the more subjects tested per day, the shorter the period. In the extreme, all members of a group could be tested at virtually the same time, and the period of testing would be very brief, as it is for one person. For epidemiologic purposes, it is often useful to describe screening programs as if all participants enter simultaneously. That is, the reference point for the determination of any measure of disease frequency in a screened population is the age at which each member enters the program, rather than the calendar time at which screening activities are begun. Persons who could have been screened but were not are considered to have entered at the age at which they became eligible for screening. If calendar time were used as a reference point, some of the changes brought about would be spread out and muted as the result of the time required to accomplish a given round of testing.

SINGLE SCREEN: In a one-time screening program, each member of a group is tested just once. By definition, no one eligible to be screened has the target disease in its clinical phase. A certain proportion of the group has preclinical disease. Which cases are actually detected depends on the sensitivity characteristics of the test and the distribution of disease manifestations. Cases diagnosed later include both false negatives and cases that did not exist or were not detectable when testing was done.

The changes in incidence rate and cumulative incidence brought about

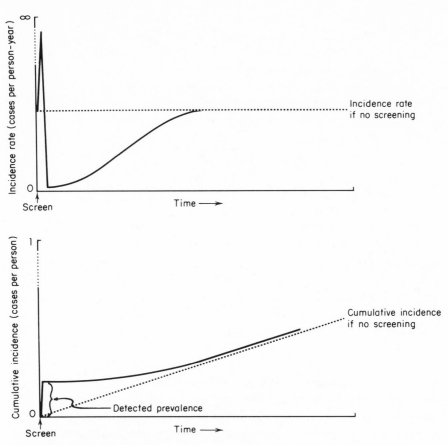

Figure 2–4. Changes in the incidence rate and cumulative incidence of a disease as a result of a single screening examination.

Source: Based on Dubin (1979).

by screening are illustrated in Figure 2–4. The curves for the screened group (solid lines) include both screen-detected cases and cases diagnosed later as a result of symptoms. The dotted lines give the expected levels of the incidence rate and cumulative incidence if no screening is done. For convenience, the expected level of the incidence rate is shown as constant. The actual rate would, however, be rising for many chronic diseases in a group as it ages with ongoing observation.

Screening converts undiagnosed disease to known disease. A rate of diagnosis for the period of screening would be very high, since the period is very brief. After screening, the incidence rate drops to a level lower than expected. The size of the deficit in incidence at a specified time after screening depends on the number of screen-detected cases that gain the corresponding amount of lead time. Some cases might be found very close to the time at which they would have caused symptoms, but other cases might be found very early in their preclinical phases, long before they normally would have been diagnosed. The shape of the curve relating incidence to time after screening is, therefore, a reflection of the distribution of lead times (Chen and Prorok, 1983).

The changes in cumulative incidence caused by screening are related to the changes in incidence rate. After the initial jump, the cumulative incidence increases more slowly than expected because of the reduced incidence rate. The expected value catches up to the observed one when the screen-detected case with the longest lead time would have been diagnosed as a result of symptoms.

Immediately after screening the prevalence of detected cases is equal to the cumulative incidence. The subsequent pattern of change in the prevalence of diagnosed disease is similar to the pattern in the cumulative incidence. However, the prevalence will generally be lower than the cumulative incidence as a result of deaths from the disease among cases, whether screen-detected or not, during the clinical phase. The prevalence would be close to the cumulative incidence near the start of screening for diseases that are not rapidly fatal.

Thus, a screening examination increases the cumulative incidence—and prevalence—of diagnosed disease and reduces the subsequent rates of diagnosis. If early diagnosis and treatment do not benefit cases by postponing or preventing the occurrence of advanced illness and death from the disease, then the rates of these events will be unchanged; the components of these rates—the number of people in the screened group at any time and the times of advanced illness or death—are not changed by early diagnosis alone.

What will happen if early treatment is beneficial? (To simplify the following discussion, only changes in the mortality rate are described. However, other measures of the value of early treatment can be used. Two examples would be the advanced illness rate, and the "quality of life" as measured by the rate of onset of disability. Changes in these measures as a result of early treatment would correspond to the indicated changes in the mortality rate.) Some of the cases detected and treated early, who otherwise would die from the disease at specific times, either have these deaths postponed or die of another cause at a later time. Deaths might be merely postponed if early treatment decreases a tumor burden but does not eradicate the disease or reduce it to the point at which the body's defenses can contain it indefinitely. The corresponding changes in mortality rate are illustrated in Figure 2–5a. Initially the rate would drop, and then it would increase when the postponed deaths occur. The mortality rate for the entire follow-

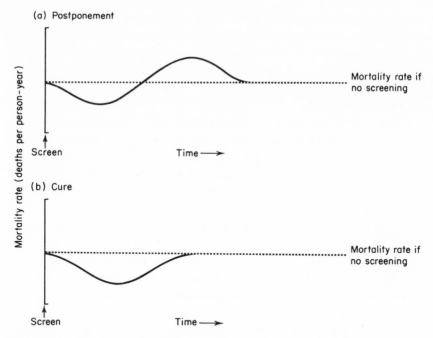

Figure 2–5. Changes in the disease-specific mortality rate brought about by postponement of death and by "cure" of screen-detected cases.

up period is reduced because cases tend to live longer, which increases the amount of person-time that they contribute to the denominator of the cause-specific death rate. The observed cumulative mortality also is reduced because some of the cases whose deaths are postponed die of other causes in the interim.

The reduction in the mortality rate from simple postponement of disease-related deaths is likely to be small unless a very long postponement is achieved. The gain would be greater if early treatment actually eradicates or cures the disease in a substantial proportion of screen-detected cases. Then, the decrease in the disease-specific mortality rate brought about by early treatment will not be offset by a later increase. The death rate in the screened group returns only to the expected level after the interval during which cured cases would have died (Figure 2–5b). (Note that, as in Figure 2–4, the expected level is shown to be constant, although it would be increasing with length of observation—ie, age—for many diseases.)

The total benefit achieved by a screening program can be expressed in several ways: the reduction in the average disease-specific mortality rate, the years of life gained (Gail, 1975), or the reduction in disease-specific cumulative mortality. All these measures are linked to the changes in mortality rate just described. The reduction in disease-specific cumulative mortality is the measure that seems to be used most often in experimental studies. The unconditional value gives the benefit in particular, practical circumstances—when the rate of all other causes of death has the value that it had in the study. The reduction in the conditional cumulative mortality is of additional scientific interest. It is what the benefit would be if people were not affected by other causes of death. The mortality rates can be used to predict what the reduction in unconditional cumulative mortality would be in various settings.[3]

Figure 2–6 illustrates relationships between changes in the natural histories of individual cases of a disease brought about by screening and early treatment, and the death rate from the disease. Each line represents the natural history of one case. A dashed line represents the portion of the preclinical phase during which the disease is undiagnosed. A dotted line represents lead time, the portion of the preclinical phase during which the disease is known as a result of screening. The clinical phase is shown by a solid line.

Suppose, first, that 20,000 people without known disease at the start are simply observed for a five-year period (Figure 2–6a). During this period, five cases of disease develop symptoms and are diagnosed, and later die, still during the period. None of the 20,000 people dies except for the five cases indicated. Therefore, the death rate from the disease in the period is

$$\text{Death rate} = \frac{5}{[(19{,}995 \times 5) + 5 + 4 + 3 + 2 + 2]\text{PY}}$$

$$= \frac{5}{99{,}991 \text{ PY}} = 5.005 \text{ per } 100{,}000 \text{ PY}$$

Now suppose that all 20,000 people are screened at the start of the observation period, but that early treatment has no effect on the progression of the disease (Figure 2–6b). Three cases—those with preclinical phases that encompass the time of testing—are detected. The other two cases could not have been detected. Since early treatment is not beneficial, the three screen-detected cases die at the same times as they would have anyway, and the natural histories of the two remaining cases are unchanged. Therefore, the screening program has no effect on the death rate.

Finally, suppose that one of the screen-detected cases is benefited by early treatment, although the other two are not (Figure 2–6c). If the case that benefits is cured and dies at some later time, of another disease, the death rate during the initial five-year period is $4/99{,}991\text{PY} = 4.004$ per

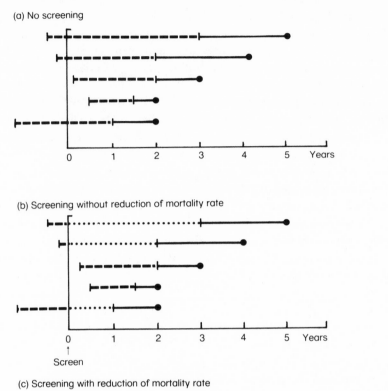

(a) No screening

(b) Screening without reduction of mortality rate

Screen

(c) Screening with reduction of mortality rate

Screen

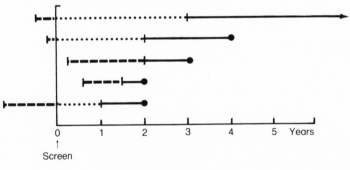

Preclinical phase (disease undiagnosed)   ▬ ▬ ▬ ▬ ▬ ▬ ▬
Lead time (asymptomatic diagnosed disease)   • • • • • • • • • • • •
Clinical phase (symptomatic diagnosed disease)   ▬▬▬▬▬▬
Death   ●

Figure 2–6. Illustration of relationships between screening and the natural history of disease.

100,000 PY, a reduction of 20%. The cumulative mortality from the disease also would be reduced by 20%. However, if death from the disease was merely postponed, the death would occur later, elevating the respective rate; the disease-specific cumulative mortality for the entire period would not be reduced.

To evaluate the efficacy of early treatment, disease-specific mortality is compared between a screened population and a similar unscreened population. If the number of screening examinations is limited (eg, a single screen, or four screens at annual intervals), it can be useful to be able to identify the groups of cases that are relevant to the effect of screening on mortality. Although the value of early treatment is limited to screen-detected cases, the groups cannot be composed of only these cases because their counterparts in the unscreened population would not be known. There would be no way to determine, for example, which three cases, and which deaths, in Figure 2–6a correspond to the experiences of the screen-detected cases in Figures 2–6b and 2–6c. Nor should these groups be defined as all cases diagnosed during an indefinitely long period after the start of observation. Cases that arise after screening is over cannot possibly be benefited by early treatment; including such cases merely obscures the value of screening. Therefore, the problem is to determine the shortest period during which the equivalent group of cases is identified in both the screened and unscreened populations. In other words, what are the temporal limits of the diagnostic effects of a screening program?

These limits can be defined in terms of cumulative incidence. The diagnostic effects of a program begin at the time of screening and can be considered to end when the cumulative incidence is the same as that in a comparable unscreened group, that is, at the time corresponding to the end of the longest lead time among screen-detected cases. This is the interval during which all screen-detected cases would have come to attention if no screening had been done. Therefore, this interval encompasses the diagnoses of all cases that could contribute to a reduction in mortality rate; cases arising later could not have been detected and treated early. In Figure 2–6, all the screen-detected cases would have been diagnosed by the end of three years after screening. The diagnostic effects of that program spanned three years; all five cases were diagnosed during that period. This definition has a drawback: The point at which the program is over may be difficult to identify with certainty. The point depends on the screening procedures used, and probably will not be able to be predicted well unless there has already been considerable experience with these procedures in the specific practical settings involved. It will usually be necessary to estimate the point of closure from the data themselves, and there may be substantial chance variability associated with the estimate. The detection of much pseudodisease creates additional complexity (see chapter 3).

To summarize, the basic information required to assess the efficacy of a given program of screening and early treatment is the time and cause of death of each case that arises while screening is having a diagnostic effect (excluding pseudodisease). If screening is beneficial, then deaths from the disease are fewer and later compared to the deaths that occur in the cases that arise in an unscreened but otherwise similar group during the equivalent time interval. In addition to the effect of early diagnosis and treatment on the natural history of the disease, the value of a screening program also depends on the mortality rate from the disease in the absence of screening, and on the mortality rate from all other causes. If the mortality rate from the disease is very low to begin with, then even an effective screening program cannot have a large arithmatic effect on the rate. If mortality from other causes is high, then a population also stands to gain little from early treatment, since cases who benefit will die soon from other causes anyway. The young would have more to gain than the old from a screening program for a disease with mortality rates that are constant with age, since young people who would otherwise die from the disease can expect to live longer than old people in whom early treatment had a similar effect on the progression of the disease. If mortality from the disease rises with age, however, more total years of life may be gained by screening older people.

REPEATED SCREENING: Suppose that a group is screened repeatedly. Typical interscreening intervals might be one to three years. As in the example of a single screen, the incidence rate and cumulative incidence increase abruptly at the initial screen. After screening, the incidence rate drops, and the increase in cumulative incidence is slower than that expected in the absence of screening. If another screening examination is done, the incidence will again rise. If the second screen is done before the end of the longest lead time among cases detected initially, the second increase in incidence (and the detected prevalence) will be smaller than the first one (if there were no false negatives, and the rate of occurrence of preclinical disease is constant). The reason for this difference is that preclinical cases removed at the first screen have not been entirely replaced when the second screen is done.

Cases with a preclinical phase of a given length will tend to be detected earlier at the second and later screens in a program than at the first one (previous false negatives aside). At the initial examination, a given case would tend to be relatively close to the time of diagnosis as a result of symptoms. If a second examination is done shortly afterward, a biologically

Table 2-1. Incidence Rates of Carcinoma of the Cervix in Connecticut, and the Percentage of Cases Diagnosed as in situ, by Year

	Incidence rate[a]			
Year	Carcinoma in situ	Invasive carcinoma	Total	Percent in situ
1950–1954	3.8	18.1	21.9	17
1955–1959	9.7	17.1	26.8	36
1960–1964	18.8	13.6	32.4	58
1965–1969	28.6	11.6	40.2	71
1970–1973	32.8	10.9	43.7	75

Source: Laskey et al (1976).
[a]Age adjusted rate per 100,000 PY.

equivalent case would be at an earlier point in the preclinical phase. If screening were nearly continuous (say, daily), then every detected case would have the maximum lead time that the screening procedure is capable of giving it. However, the therapeutic value of the additional lead time from repeated as compared to one-time screening is not known for any chronic disease.

If screening, once begun, is continued indefinitely, the average incidence rate of the disease increases. The most important reason for such an increase would usually be the detection of nonprogressive cases. In Connecticut, the sum of the age-adjusted incidence rates of noninvasive and invasive carcinoma of the cervix was 21.9 per 100,000 PY in 1950–1954, and 43.7 in 1970–1973 (Table 2–1) (Laskey et al, 1976). This increase is attributable entirely to an increasing rate of carcinoma in situ. The close relation of the increasing use of the Pap smear to the overall rise in incidence suggests that it is largely the result of the detection of cases that would not cause symptoms. This pseudodisease is, arguably, a reasonable price to pay for the control of cervical cancer by screening. By advancing the time of diagnosis of progressive cases, screening tends to increase incidence rates at low ages with a compensatory decrease at higher ages. In principle, continuous screening also increases the overall incidence rate by reducing the person-time that cases contribute to the denominator of the rate (Morrison, 1979a). In practice, however, this effect is unlikely to be important. Therefore, established repetitive screening has little influence on the incidence rate of a disease in which all, or nearly all, cases are progressive.

As pointed out at the beginning of this book, the earliness of diagnosis may be affected by unplanned changes in medical practice or medical awareness, as well as by intentional screening. In recent decades, there have been increases in the incidence rates of cancers of the breast, large intestine, and prostate. These increases have been rapid and in some cases, irregular, and not accompanied by corresponding increases in mortality. One explanation of these increases is heightened concern over the possibility of cancer, an increasingly vigorous search for abnormal masses, and an increasing tendency to diagnose as malignant lesions previously considered benign (Doll and Peto, 1981).

NOTES

[1] In this book, the CFR is defined as having a person-time denominator. The term *case-fatality rate* has been used elsewhere to describe the proportion of cases that die within some period after diagnosis. Here, this proportion is defined as the cumulative case fatality.

[2] Let $M_{i,d}$ be the mortality rate from the disease of interest during the ith time interval Δt_i, and let $Q_{c,T}$ be the conditional cumulative mortality from the start of observation through time T. Then,

$$Q_{c,T} = 1 - \exp\left(-\sum_{i=1}^{T} M_{i,d} \, \Delta t_i\right)$$

The conditional cumulative incidence is derived in the same way, with incidence rates substituted for mortality rates.

[3] Let $M_{i,d}$ be the mortality rate from the disease of interest, $M_{i,+}$ the death rate from all causes, $q_{i,u}$ the unconditional cumulative mortality during Δt_i, and $Q_{u,T}$ the unconditional cumulative mortality from the start of observation through the time T. Then,

$$q_{u,i} = \frac{M_{i,d}}{M_{i,+}} \left[1 - \exp\left(-M_{i,+} \, \Delta t_i\right)\right]$$

and

$$Q_{u,T} = \prod_{i=1}^{T} (1 - q_{u,i})$$

3 Early Detection: Sensitivity and Lead Time

For any screening program to be successful at reducing morbidity or mortality, a substantial proportion of cases must be detected during the preclinical phase with enough lead time for treatment to be more effective than it would be if it were not done early. *Sensitivity* is the property of a test that enables cases to be detected early. The sensitivity characteristics of a test also determine the lead times that detected cases gain. Because of the close connection between sensitivity and lead time, both topics are discussed in this chapter, and the relation of the sensitivity characteristics of a test to the lead-time distribution is described.

Another important property of a screening test is its *specificity*. The specificity describes the ability of a test to identify nondiseased people. Because both sensitivity and specificity must be adequate for a test to be useful, they are often considered together, as in chapter 1. However, these measures refer to fundamentally different aspects of test performance. Sensitivity is an important determinant of the disease-control value of a program. In contrast, the specificity has a major influence on costs and feasibility. Therefore, sensitivity and specificity are dealt with separately, specificity being addressed in chapter 7.

SENSITIVITY

The sensitivity of an analytic procedure generally is described in terms of the amount or concentration of a substance which that procedure is capable of detecting. For example, the Hemoccult test has been found to be positive on most applications only if the stool contains at least 8 to 10 mg hemoglobin per gram, which would be the result of the loss of about 10 ml blood per day in the large intestine (Ostrow, 1979; Stroehlein, 1979).

Modern mammography can detect tumors that are less than 1 cm in diameter (Alexander et al, 1990; Silverstein et al, 1989). Since the purpose of screening is to enable cases of disease to be treated early, rather than to find blood, masses, or other manifestations for their own sake, another definition of sensitivity has evolved in the screening context. The sensitivity of a screening test is, therefore, usually defined as

$$\text{Sensitivity} = \frac{\text{Number with preclinical disease who are positive on test}}{\text{Total number tested who have preclinical disease}}$$

$$(3-1)$$

This definition is linked to the more general idea of sensitivity through the numerator of (3–1), which depends on the number in whom the disease manifestation tested for is present at a high enough level to be detected. The detected cases are termed *true positives*. Cases of disease with a negative test result are designated *false negatives*.

The presence of preclinical disease may be defined by the same manifestation as that on which the screening test is based. Diabetes is a good example (Thorner and Remein, 1967). Suppose that a large number of people without known diabetes are tested by means of the glucose tolerance test—a *diagnostic* test for the disease. Individuals positive to this test are considered to have preclinical diabetes. Suppose that 150 such people are found. These people might then be tested by the "random" blood sugar method—a *screening* test for diabetes. If 34 of these people had values of at least 180 mg/100 ml and thus were positive to the screening test, its sensitivity would be estimated as 34/150 = 23%.

On the other hand, diagnostic and screening tests may be based on quite different manifestations of preclinical disease. Ultrasound examination is an accurate diagnostic test for fetal anencephaly. The level of alpha-feto-protein (AFP) in maternal serum may be used as a screening test for the condition. The test is usually done early in the second trimester of pregnancy. The test is considered to be positive if the level is at least 2.5 times the median value for a given gestational age in women with unaffected pregnancies. The sensitivity of the AFP test is estimated to be 88% (Wald and Cuckle, 1987).

The definition of sensitivity given by expression (3–1) is complicated by conceptual and practical difficulties. One problem is that the level of the manifestation of a disease—blood, mass, etc—that causes a positive test might not be readily defined for individuals. The likelihood that a cytologic test for cancer is positive, for example, might be roughly proportional to the rate at which cells are exfoliated (ie, the number of cells that are shed per unit time), rather than being essentially zero for tumors with low rates and 100% for those with higher rates. If so, it might not be possible to determine, by a means other than the test itself, whether a given case ought to appear in the numerator of the sensitivity, that is, whether a case would be detected by screening. Some cases, perhaps most, might have a probability of detection that is not at either extreme. Thus, the sensitivity of the test would correspond to the average probability of detection of a group of tumors with a distribution of rates of exfoliation.

Another problem is that the denominator of the sensitivity—the total number tested who have preclinical disease—must inevitably be determined by tests that constitute a diagnostic procedure. Like screening tests, diagnostic tests are subject to errors, and one diagnostic procedure may, in fact, be more sensitive than another. A given screening test would appear relatively sensitive if compared to a relatively insensitive diagnostic test. Therefore, any estimate of sensitivity should be regarded as the sensitivity of one test (the screening test) relative to another (the diagnostic test), rather than as a value with any absolute meaning.

Finally, and most important in practice, it may not be medically acceptable to identify people with early disease by a method that is independent of the screening test to be evaluated. Diagnostic tests for cancer usually involve surgery and would not be done on someone who is asymptomatic and without any other indication of the presence of disease. In such circumstances, the denominator for an estimate of sensitivity cannot be determined directly.

After a new test has been developed, it is important to decide whether its sensitivity is high enough to consider using it in a screening program, or whether the test needs to be further refined, or perhaps abandoned. Preliminary estimates of sensitivity may be obtained by testing patients who have already been definitively diagnosed with the disease. Testing patients avoids the problem of applying a diagnostic test to well people. Furthermore, this approach is a natural outgrowth of the fact that screening tests often are modifications of procedures developed for diagnostic purposes. Sensitivity data derived from symptomatic patients must, however, be viewed with caution, because a test's sensitivity is likely to be higher, perhaps much higher, in cases with symptomatic disease than in cases with the preclinical condition. If it is necessary to obtain preliminary information on sensitivity by testing patients, rather than asymptomatic people, it is best to do this as close to the time of initial diagnosis as possible. This goal may be achieved by using the test under consideration, along with established procedures, for differential diagnosis. Farrow (1979) compared the result of urine cytology as a test for bladder cancer to the final diagnosis of patients attending a urology outpatient department (Table 3–1). In this group, 1310 patients ultimately were found to have bladder cancer. If patients with malignant cytology are considered positive, the sensitivity is

Table 3–1. Relation of Urine Cytology Testing and Final Diagnosis in Urologic Outpatients

Final diagnosis	Result of cytology			Total
	Malignant	Atypical	Negative	
Bladder cancer	692	180	438	1,310
No bladder cancer	92	228	8,596	8,916

Source: Farrow GM: Pathologist's role in bladder cancer. *Semin Oncol* 1978: 6:198–206. Reprinted by permission of Grune & Stratton, Inc.

estimated as $692/1,310 = 53\%$. If atypical cytology is considered positive as well, the sensitivity would be $(692 + 180)/1,310 = 67\%$. In either case, these estimates are likely to be somewhat high compared to what they would be if asymptomatic people were screened. The sensitivity of a test might also appear high in a population that is normally subject to a relatively low level of medical care. Such a population will have a relatively high proportion of advanced, although undiagnosed, cases.

Often, the desired information on sensitivity can only be obtained in actual screening circumstances. Would the additional use of mammography find more cases at a given screen than would be found in a breast cancer screening program based only on physical examination? This question cannot be answered by investigating symptomatic patients since they virtually all have palpable tumors. However, answers have been furnished by breast cancer screening programs. For instance, investigators at the Health Insurance Plan of Greater New York (HIP) conducted an experimental trial of screening for breast cancer that began in the 1960s (Shapiro et al, 1988). This study was described briefly in chapter 1, and the methods and results are presented in detail in the next chapter. The Breast Cancer Detection Demonstration Project (BCDDP) was a nonexperimental screening activity carried out in 27 sites in the United States during the the 1970s. About 250,000 women age 35 to 74 were enrolled in a program of five annual screening examinations (Baker, 1982). Both the HIP and BCDDP programs included physical and mammographic examinations of the breast.

Table 3–2 shows the percentages of screen-detected cases of breast cancer according to the type of test. In the HIP study, 67% of cases were detected by physical examination (including cases also detected by mammography) and 55% were detected by mammography (including cases also detected by physical examination). Thus, physical examination appeared somewhat more sensitive. Mammography alone, however, accounted for one-third of the screen-detected cases, so this procedure did appear to make a substantial contribution to case detection.

Table 3-2. Percentages of Screen-detected Cases of Breast Cancer in the HIP Study and the BCDDP that Were Detected by Physical Examination and by Mammography

	Type of examination		
	Physical examination only	Mammography only	Physical examination and mammography
HIP	45%	33%	22%
BCDDP	9	42	49

Sources: Shapiro et al (1988)—HIP data; Baker (1982)—BCDDP data.

A decade of improvements in mammography technique is generally considered to be the main reason for the large difference between the HIP and BCDDP figures. In the latter study, 58% of cases were detected by physical examination, but 91% were detected by mammography. That is, mammography appeared 1.57 times as sensitive as physical examination, and physical examination alone accounted for only 9% of screen-detected cases.

Thermography is another procedure that can be used to detect breast cancer. A cancerous breast tends to have a higher skin temperature than the opposite breast does; these temperature differences are visualized by thermography. Compared to mammography, the advantages of thermography are lower cost and lack of any radiation hazard. Preliminary studies were made of the sensitivity and specificity of thermography compared to mammography and physical examination in the diagnosis of symptomatic breast cancer. Lilienfeld et al (1969) conducted a large study and found that the sensitivities (and specificities) of the three techniques were similar. Thermography was subsequently evaluated in the BCDDP, where the findings left doubt as to its usefulness in screening (Beahrs et al, 1979). Initially, subjects in the BCDDP were examined by thermography as well as mammography and physical examination. At the first screening examination, about 41% of all breast cancers found were positive by thermography. In contrast, 92% of these cases were positive by mammography, and 55% were positive by physical examination. Thus, the sensitivity of thermography was less than half that of mammography, and about three-fourths that of physical examination. Moreover, about 29% of the cases identified in the first examination were detected by mammography only; these would not have been found if thermography had been substituted for mammography in the screening procedure. Of minimal cancers (non-invasive or <1 cm in diameter), 37% were detected by mammography alone. As a result of these findings, thermography was discontinued in the BCDDP. (The BCDDP did not present data on the specificity of thermography, but findings in a screening project in Sweden suggest that the specificity may be as low as 50% (Minutes, 1982).)

The sensitivity data just given on physical examination, mammography, and thermography are based on comparisons of the proportion of known cases detected by each of the tests. These proportions do not correspond to the sensitivity of the test as defined by expression (3–1), since some cases of preclinical disease may have remained undetected. However, data from screening programs also have been used to obtain rough estimates of the actual sensitivity without applying diagnostic tests to large numbers of well people. The approach that has been used is to treat interval cases—those that come to attention with symptoms soon after a negative screening examination—as false negatives; it is assumed that interval cases were in the preclinical phase at the time of screening. In a study in Malmo, Sweden, for example, 8 cases of breast cancer were detected by screening with physical examination; within the next year, 10 more cases were diagnosed in women who had screened negative. The sensitivity of physical examination would be estimated as $8/18 = 44\%$ (Lundgren, 1979). In the HIP study, 132 cases were found by screening, and 47 more were diagnosed in the year following a negative test (Shapiro et al, 1988). The sensitivity would be estimated as 74%; this is the value for screening with *both* mammography and physical examination. Separate estimates of this type for the two procedures cannot be obtained from the HIP study because both procedures were used on all women who were screened.

The validity of estimating sensitivity using interval cases is uncertain. It usually is not possible to distinguish interval cases that were truly false negatives from newly detectable cases with short preclinical phases that had not begun at the time of testing. Moreover, the findings obviously depend on the length of the follow-up interval selected.

The interval case approach suggests a quantity that might be called the *program sensitivity,* which can be defined as the proportion of cases found as a result of screening among all cases that arise during a screening program (Morrison, 1985). In contrast to the sensitivity as defined in expression (3–1), the denominator of the program sensitivity is likely to include symptomatic, as well as asymptomatic, cases. In order to determine the program sensitivity, it is necessary to observe the screened group during the period of time over which the diagnostic effects of screening are felt. The detection of pseudodisease affects the program sensitivity. As shown in this chapter, however, the amount of pseudodisease can be estimated, and measures of program sensitivity can be derived that exclude pseudodisease (Day, 1985; Chamberlain et al, 1986).

The program sensitivity depends on both the sensitivity of the test in use and the frequency of screening; shorter intervals between examinations increase the proportion of screen-detected cases. In the HIP study, the diagnostic effects of screening appeared to end about five years after the experiment began; the numbers of breast cancers diagnosed in the screened and unscreened groups became approximately equal at that time (pages 58 to 60). Of the 304 cases diagnosed in the screened group, 132 were detected early. Therefore, the program sensitivity is estimated as 132/304 or 43%. There were 225 cases diagnosed during the first five years in the group that was screened at least once. Based on participants, therefore, the program sensitivity is estimated as 132/225 = 59%.

The program sensitivity can only be high for diseases in which the duration of the preclinical phase tends to be long in relation to the interval between screening examinations. If the preclinical phase is short and the interval between examinations is long, only a small fraction of cases can be detected. This is one reason that screening is potentially useful in the control of chronic but not acute diseases; the preclinical phase of acute diseases is too short for the program sensitivity to be high unless screening is done very often.

The program sensitivity can be predicted without the need for prolonged follow-up if there is some advance knowledge of the nature of the distribution of the duration of preclinical disease (Day, 1985). This distribution, however, depends on the test in use. Adequate knowledge of the distribution associated with a new test may not be available to make an accurate prediction of its program sensitivity.

In some circumstances, the program sensitivity will be about equal to the sensitivity as defined conventionally. This will be true if every preclinical case is tested and there is no pseudodisease. Prenatal screening for neural tube defects or Down syndrome with 100% participation meets these criteria.

Finally, the sensitivity of a test is sometimes defined with respect to the serious outcome—disability or death—to be prevented. This issue is considered further in chapter 7.

LEAD TIME

A case that is detected by screening experiences lead time from detection up to the time at which diagnosis would have occurred without screening (Hutchison and Shapiro, 1968). Except for any effects of screening or early treatment, however, such a case would not have symptoms related to the disease during the lead-time interval, and the existence of the disease would not otherwise be known.

The lead time gained by screening may vary substantially from case to case. If detection occurs just before clinical diagnosis would, then the lead time for that case is very short. On the other hand, if detection occurs early in the preclinical phase, the lead time is relatively long. People who have nonprogressive disease (pseudodisease) that is detected experience lead-time intervals that are indefinitely long.

Pathologic characteristics indicative of early disease may reflect lead time. In the HIP breast cancer study, for example, 71% of screen-detected cases were in the localized stage at the time of diagnosis, but only 46% were localized in the unscreened control group (Shapiro et al, 1988). There has been a large increase in the proportion of cases of cervical cancer diagnosed in the noninvasive, in situ stage since the 1950s (Table 2–1). This trend is the result of lead time gained by increasing use of the Pap smear. As mentioned in chapter 2, much of this lead time may result from the detection of nonprogressive disease.

In most circumstances it is impossible to determine the lead times experienced by individual cases. To do this would require that people be screened, and those found to have the disease not be treated nor even informed of the findings. The time at which diagnosis and treatment as a result of symptoms ultimately occurs in each of these people would be related to the time of detection by screening to give the lead time. In practice, of course, people who have screen-detected disease have some sort of treatment. At a minimum, they are informed that they have a condition that should be evaluated from time to time. It cannot be reasonably assumed in either instance that symptoms would appear when they would have if the disease had not been detected early. Early treatment, if successful, would prevent or postpone symptoms. On the other hand, a patient's knowledge of a diagnosis might lead to heightened awareness and the appearance of symptoms earlier than otherwise. The lead times of individual cases can, however, be predicted in prenatal screening for conditions such as neural tube defects or Down syndrome, since the conditions would be diagnosed at birth in the absence of screening.

Although lead time generally cannot be determined for individual cases, it *is* possible to measure the lead-time distribution—the numbers of screen-detected cases that gain specified amounts of lead time. Knowledge of the lead time gained by screening is valuable for several reasons. First, it helps to give some idea of the length of time by which treatment must be advanced in order to achieve a particular reduction in morbidity or mortality. The lead-time distribution also may suggest the distribution of the duration of the preclinical phase. The latter distribution is an important aspect of the natural history of a disease and it may be useful in planning screening programs. Furthermore, information on lead time is useful for interpreting the observed clinical course of cases detected by screening (chapter 6). Finally, the lead-time distribution depends on the sensitivity characteristics of the screening test used, and various measures of sensitivity can be related to this distribution. It should be kept in mind that lead time is measured chronologically and the biological significance of a given amount of lead time may differ from case to case; a given lead time may vary as to the proportion of the total preclinical phase that it represents, and the value of treatment advanced by a given amount of lead time may vary from one case to another.

The hypothetical data given in Figure 2–6 provide a simple illustration of a lead-time distribution. This figure shows what the natural histories of five cases might be in a population that is, or is not, subjected to a one-time screening program. If there is no screening, the five cases would be diagnosed at times 1, 1½, 2, 2, and 3 years after the start of observation. If, on the other hand, the population is screened once, three cases would be detected by screening (at the start of observation); the remaining two cases would be diagnosed at 1½ and 2 years as a result of symptoms.

The differences in the times of diagnosis with and without screening are the lead times. By comparing the times of diagnosis of cases in the screened and unscreened populations, it is apparent that the three screen-detected cases would have been diagnosed at 1, 2, and 3 years after the start of observation if screening had not been done. Thus, the lead times gained by these cases are 1, 2, and 3 years. During the first year after screening all three cases experience lead time, during the second year, two cases experience lead time, and during the third year, one case experiences lead time. This information is summarized conveniently by Figure 3–1, which gives one form of the distribution of lead time:

The proportion of cases detected with lead time > 0 year $= 1$.
The proportion of cases detected with lead time > 1 year $= \frac{2}{3}$.
The proportion of cases detected with lead time > 2 years $= \frac{1}{3}$.
The proportion of cases detected with lead time > 3 years $= 0$.

The proportions of cases having lead time in a given interval can be determined from this cumulative distribution by repeated subtraction:

The proportion of cases with lead time > 0 year and ≤ 1 year $= \frac{1}{3}$.
The proportion of cases with lead time > 1 year and ≤ 2 years $= \frac{1}{3}$.
The proportion of cases with lead time > 2 years and ≤ 3 years $= \frac{1}{3}$.

In this example, the only changes in the number of cases experiencing lead time occur abruptly at the end of the first, second, and third years of observation. Therefore, the fact that there is one case each with a lead time of exactly one, two, and three years can be deduced from Figure 3–1. Nor-

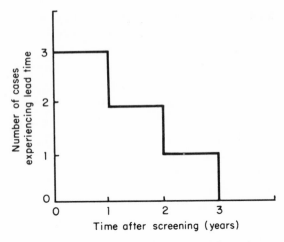

Figure 3–1. Example of a lead-time distribution: number of cases experiencing lead time by time after screening.

mally, the distribution of lead times would have to be related to a series of time categories as above.

The total lead time generated by the screening program is equal to the area contained by the distribution in Figure 3–1. This area is (3 cases × 1 year) + (2 cases × 1 year) + (1 case × 1 year) = 6 case-years. The average lead time experienced by a screen-detected case is, then,

$$\frac{6 \text{ case-years}}{3 \text{ cases}} = 2 \text{ years}$$

As noted above, it would normally not be possible to tell which case gained a specific amount of lead time. Even so, the numbers of cases that experience lead times within specified limits can be determined by comparing the curve of the cumulative number of cases diagnosed according to time in the screened population to the curve for an unscreened population that was otherwise identical. The lower portion of Figure 2–4 is a general example of such curves. Figure 3–2 is an illustration that is derived from Figure 2–6. The distribution of the area between the curves in Figure 3–2 corresponds to the distribution of the lead time given in Figure 3–1. Thus, the distribution of lead time can be defined as the distribution of *excess case-time* created by early detection. The lead-time distribution is the distribution of exposure to the earliness of treatment that screening brings about.

Now consider the measurement of lead time in more general terms (Hutchison and Shapiro, 1968; Morrison, 1982b). Imagine a population without cases of clinical disease that is screened once. Detected cases that

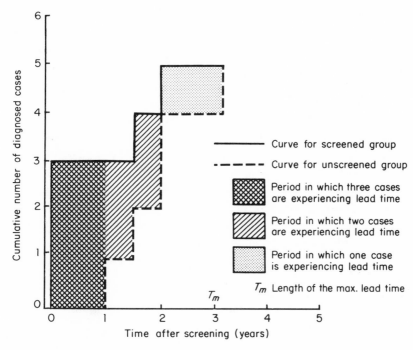

Figure 3–2. Example of estimation of lead-time distribution by comparison of cumulative numbers of cases diagnosed in screened and unscreened groups.

are confirmed by diagnostic tests have disease that is in the preclinical phase. All cases discovered are treated, and no further screening is done. The screened persons enter observation at the time of screening. For persons who refuse screening, observation begins when screening would have been done. Cases of clinically diagnosed illness are treated as they arise. For comparison, imagine a population identical to that offered screening. This population enters observation at the same time as the screened population, but is not screened. As cases become symptomatic they are identified and treated. For simplicity, the screened and unscreened populations are taken to be the same size. If they are not, adjustment can readily be made by applying the appropriate proportionality factor.

In the screened population let

C_{0s} = number of cases detected by the screening examination
$C_{i.}$ = total number of diagnosed cases at time i after entry, whether or not these cases were detected by screening

In the unscreened population let

$\overline{C}_i$ = total number of diagnosed cases at time i after entry

C_i and $\overline{C}_i$ can be defined as either the cumulative numbers diagnosed or the prevalent numbers remaining alive. Estimation of a lead-time distribution is somewhat simpler when based on the cumulative numbers and this approach is used in the present chapter. However, the analysis of the clinical course of screen-detected disease, given in chapter 6, is based on the prevalent numbers.[1]

Suppose that time after the start of the study is divided into intervals of constant length that are designated Δt. The number of cases experiencing lead time during a given interval is approximated by the corresponding value of $C_i - \overline{C}_i$. The prevalent number experiencing lead time during an interval will be nearly equal to the difference in the respective cumulative numbers diagnosed as long as the death rate from all causes is low and not too much time has elapsed after screening. If early treatment is effective, the excess number of prevalent cases in the screened group must be reduced by the number alive for this reason. This issue is considered further in chapter 6.

The number of cases experiencing lead time is greatest just after screening, when the only diagnosed cases are the screen-detected ones. The number experiencing lead time decreases with the passage of time as the counterparts of screen-detected cases are diagnosed clinically in the unscreened group. The number of diagnosed cases in the screened group exceeds the number in the unscreened group until the time at which the end of the preclinical phase has been reached for all screen-detected cases.

The relative numbers of cases that experience lead times of specified durations give the lead-time distribution. The number of cases that have a lead time of at least i is $l_i = C_i - \overline{C}_i$ (provided that the true incidence of the disease is not affected by screening (J. Emerson, Ph.D., oral communication, 1984)). The proportion of all screen-detected cases that have a lead time (L) at least as great as i is

$$Pr(L \geq i) = \frac{l_i}{C_{0s}} \tag{3-2}$$

Expression (3–2) is one minus the observed cumulative distribution function of the lead time. Note that cases among people who decline to be screened, as well as false negatives that are diagnosed later, make no contribution to the lead time. The lead time is derived entirely from true positives.

The proportion of screen-detected cases that experiences lead time at least as great as i, but less than $i + \Delta t$, is readily estimated by subtraction:

$$Pr(i \leq L < i + \Delta t) = \frac{l_i - l_{i+\Delta t}}{C_{0s}} \tag{3-3}$$

Expression (3–3) is the observed probability distribution function of the lead time. Chen and Prorok (1983) derived the p.d.f. of the lead time from the difference, by time, between the incidence rate after entry in a screened group and a comparable unscreened group (Figure 2–4, upper portion). The excess cases diagnosed in the unscreened group in a given time interval are the counterparts of screen-detected cases that had lead times approximately equal to the time from entry to the midpoint of the selected interval. Therefore, the relative sizes of the differences in incidence in each interval give the relative numbers of cases with the corresponding lead time.

The total observed lead time is the area between two curves similar to those in Figure 3–2. The amount of lead time experienced during one interval is the number of cases, l_i, multiplied by the width of the interval, Δt, or $l_i \, \Delta t$. L_{tot}, the total lead time—the total case-time created by early detection—is equal to the sum of these area elements beginning at the time of screening and ending at the time that the curves meet, or T_m. T_m is the length of the maximum lead time experienced by a screen-detected case. At T_m, the prevalence of cases in the screened and unscreened groups are equal, and after T_m there are no cases experiencing lead time.

$$L_{tot} = \sum_{i < T_m} l_i \, \Delta t \tag{3–4}$$

The mean lead time, $\overline{L}$, is obtained by dividing L_{tot} by C_{0s}.

$$\overline{L} = \frac{L_{tot}}{C_{0s}} \tag{3–5}$$

The value obtained in (3–5) is the average lead time for screen-detected cases. Cases that are not detected by screening do not gain any lead time. Therefore, the mean lead time gained by all cases diagnosed in the course of the screening program, whether or not they are screen-detected, is equal to $\overline{L}$ multiplied by the proportion of all cases in the program that were screen-detected. If the number of cases coming to attention in the entire program is C_{T_m}, the mean lead time gained by these cases is $(C_{0s}/C_{T_m})\overline{L}$.

At T_m, the purely diagnostic effect of a screening program is over. As pointed out in chapter 2, it may be difficult to identify this time precisely. Moreover, T_m may be many years long if disease in the preclinical phase progresses slowly, and T_m can never be observed if screening detects more than a negligible amount of pseudodisease. If T_m in a program has not yet been reached, the total and mean values for the lead time cannot be obtained. Once there have been i years of observation, however, the lead-time distribution up to time i (expressions (3–2) and (3–3)) can be estimated.

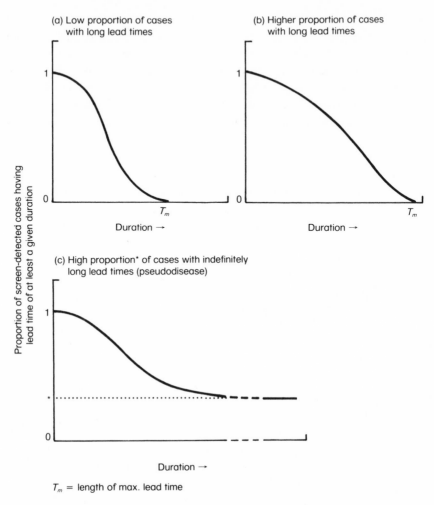

T_m = length of max. lead time

Figure 3–3. Illustrations of different types of lead-time distributions.

Figure 3–3 illustrates three different cumulative lead-time distributions. Part (a) shows a small proportion of cases with a long lead time. Part (b) shows a relatively high proportion of cases with a long lead time. Part (c) shows a lead-time distribution that might be observed if screening detects pseudodisease as well as disease that would progress to cause clinical illness. Dunn (1953) posed the question as to what percentage of carcinoma in situ of the cervix ultimately becomes invasive. The general issue is whether, and to what extent, minimal disease detected by screening is pseudodisease that would not progress, in contrast to real disease that is detected early. The amount of pseudodisease may be estimated from the asymptotic value of the lead-time distribution as indicated by the broken horizontal line, (Figure 3–3(c)). This value is reached at the time that the curves of cumulative incidence in the screened group and an otherwise similar unscreened group become parallel permanently. This is also the point at which the incidence rates in the two groups become the same. The time at which the asymptotic value is reached corresponds to T_m in the absence of pseudodisease. If there is pseudodisease, the lead-time distribution has components attributable to pseudodisease and to progressive disease.

The fact that the lead time created by screening can be influenced strongly by the detection of pseudodisease reinforces the inappropriateness of viewing lead time (or other diagnostic effects) as a measure of the ultimate success of a screening program. The lead time might be very high only as a result of the diagnosis of disease that would never become clinical and would never require treatment.

REPEATED SCREENING EXAMINATIONS: So far, the discussion has concerned the lead time generated by a single screening examination. What happens if a screening program consists of repeated examinations? If the screening is done at intervals greater than T_m, then the lead-time distribution for each screen may be evaluated separately as described above. From the diagnostic point of view, each round of screening would constitute a distinct program. Typically, however, rescreening is done at intervals shorter than T_m to ensure detection of a substantial proportion of cases. Since the screening is done at relatively short intervals, some cases detected at one examination continue to experience lead time after a subsequent examination. Consequently, it would not be known whether a case diagnosed in the unscreened population corresponds to a case diagnosed at an earlier or a later examination in the screened population and it would not be possible to identify the number of cases experiencing lead time as the result of a specific examination once another one has occurred. Therefore, the distributions given by (3–2) and (3–3) can only be estimated for the portion of the program from the first to the second screen. However, the total and mean lead time created by the entire screening program can be evaluated using expressions (3–4) and (3–5) provided that the screening examinations do not continue indefinitely. As in the case of a program with a single screening examination, l_i is the difference in the frequency of diagnosed cases between the screened and unscreened populations at time i after the start of the program. The quantity C_{0s} is taken to be the total number of cases detected by all screening examinations. T_m is taken to be that time after the start of the screening program at which the numbers of diagnosed cases in the screened and unscreened groups become equal after the last examination.

It would be possible to estimate the complete lead-time distribution for each one of several examinations if information were available for comparable populations screened exactly once, twice, three times, etc, and not at all. The lead-time distribution for the first examination would be estimated as described above using data on the population screened only once, and data on the unscreened population. The distribution for the second examination would be derived from a comparison of the group screened twice to the group screened only once. In other words, expressions (3–2) and (3–3) would apply, with the group screened twice taken as the "screened population" and the group screened once being taken as the "unscreened population." A corresponding procedure could be applied to subsequent examinations.

The estimation of lead-time functions in a program of multiple screening examinations is illustrated with data drawn from one such program, the HIP study (Shapiro et al, 1988). The data are presented in Table 3–3

Table 3–3. Estimation of Total and Mean Lead Time in HIP Study

	Completed year after entry (j)						
	1	2	3	4	5	6	7
Study group							
a. Cases detected by screening during the year	54	31	20	25	2	0	0
b. Total cases diagnosed during the year	79	60	49	62	54	63	59
c. Cumulative number of cases diagnosed by end of the year	79	139	188	250	304	367	426
d. Average number of diagnosed cases during the year (C_j)	48.4	113.8	165.1	219.8	277.0	337.4	396.1
Control group							
e. Cases diagnosed during the year	59	65	40	55	79	70	76
f. Cumulative number of cases diagnosed by the end of the year	59	124	164	219	298	368	444
g. Average number of diagnosed cases during the year (C_j)	31.1	92.4	144.3	193.1	261.1	331.0	407.0
Number of cases experiencing lead time (d–g) during the year (l_j)	17.3	21.4	20.8	26.7	15.9	6.4	−10.9

Total lead time based on first five years = L_{tot} = (17.3 + 21.4 + 20.8 + 26.7 + 15.9) × 1 year = 102.1 years.

Mean lead time based on first five years = $\bar{L}$ = 102.1 years/(54 + 31 + 20 + 25 + 2) = 0.77 years = 9.3 months.

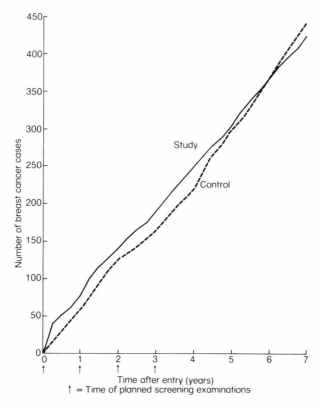

Figure 3–4. Cumulative numbers of cases of breast cancer diagnosed by time in the HIP study.

and Figure 3–4. For convenience, the time of diagnosis of each case was considered to be the midpoint of the respective quarter-year after entry. Thus, the maximum difference between the actual and assumed dates of diagnosis was 6½ weeks. The numbers of diagnosed cases in the screened and unscreened groups at time i after entry, C_i and $\overline{C}_i$, are expressed in Table 3–3 as averages over periods of a year. In the study group, the number of diagnosed cases increases abruptly at the start of the study, again at the start of the second year, and more slowly between examinations with the addition of interval cases. In the control group, the number of cases increases regularly with time after the start of observation.

Although the screening examinations were planned to be done at annual intervals, there were delays in some of the examinations or in the completion of diagnostic studies in women who screened positive. As a result, the diagnosis of some screen-detected cases occurred months after the planned time of the screening examinations. There were 54 screen-detected cases diagnosed in the first year of the study. Of these, 34 were diagnosed in the first quarter-year, 10 in the second quarter-year, 4 in the third, and 6 in the fourth. The cumulative effect of these delays in examinations and subsequent diagnosis increased as the study progressed. Thus, there were 20 screen-detected cases diagnosed in the third year of the study. The numbers diagnosed in successive quarter-years were 7, 4, 7, and 2. Delays in diagnosis reduce the lead time compared to what it would have been if all diagnoses of screen-detected cases had occurred close to the planned times of the screening examinations. Through the first four years of the program, the cumulative number of diagnosed cases in the study group (Table 3–3, line c) clearly exceeds the number in the control group (line f). The difference between the two groups was small from the end of the fifth year on. (This result indicates that the program detected little or no pseudodisease.) Therefore, it might be assumed, perhaps with some error, that T_m occurs at the end of the fifth year ($i = 5$). The total lead time is then estimated as

$$L_{tot} = \sum_{i=1}^{5} l_i \, \Delta t = (17.3 + 21.4 + 20.8 + 26.7 + 15.9) \times 1 \text{ yr}$$

$$= 102.1 \text{ years}$$

Since 132 cases (all cases in line a in Table 3–3) were detected by the four screening examinations, the mean lead time experienced by these cases is estimated as

$$\overline{L} = \frac{L_{tot}}{C_{0s}} = \frac{102.1 \text{ years}}{132} = 0.77 \text{ years}$$

The lead-time distribution of cases diagnosed at the first examination could be evaluated using expressions (3–2) and (3–3) only for the first 12 months of the program, that is, until the second screen. The lead time experienced during this period would, of course, be less than the total lead time experienced during the entire program. A method is presented in chapter 5 to estimate the effect of a specified schedule of screening on mortality among persons who comply with the schedule. This method also may be used to estimate the lead-time distribution experienced by persons who comply with the schedule.

THE RELATION OF SENSITIVITY AND LEAD TIME

It is useful to define the sensitivity of a test by its relation to the lead-time distribution. The determination of a lead-time distribution does not depend on widespread application of a diagnostic test; the role of the diagnostic test is only to confirm a positive screening test. Differences in the lead-time distributions generated by various tests applied to similar populations must reflect differences in the sensitivity characteristics of the tests, in particular, differences in the way in which the probability of detection by each test changes as the preclinical phase progresses.

First consider the detection of an individual case. The probability that a case is positive on a test (the detectability of the case) depends on the point in the preclinical phase at which screening is done. The detectability is equivalent to what the sensitivity of the test would be for a group of identical cases with a given degree of the manifestation tested for. Very early in the preclinical phase, the disease will not be detectable. The detectability will tend to increase as the preclinical phase progresses, but different patterns of increase are possible. For example, detectability might depend strongly on whether or not a lesion bleeds or has attained a certain size. Detectability would then increase rapidly as this state is reached, and subsequently increase very little. A pattern of this type might be characteristic of the Hemoccult test for colonic bleeding, or the detection of a mass by physical or x-ray examination, but such a pattern might not occur generally. The probability of a positive cytology test for cancer was suggested above to be proportional to the rate at which cells are exfoliated. This rate might increase gradually, with the surface area of the tumor, and without any sudden jumps. In any event, the proportion of a group of preclinical cases that would be expected to be detected is equal to their *average* probability of detection at the time of testing. In practice, only the numerator of this proportion—the number of cases detected—can be determined; the denominator is the total number of cases in the preclinical phase and this quantity could be known only if a perfect diagnostic test were available and could be applied. If the denominator were known, however, the proportion would be the observed value of the true sensitivity.

The change in the detectability of each case as the disease progresses suggests the idea of a *sensitivity function* (Eddy, 1980)—sensitivity according to the point in the preclinical phase at which cases are tested. Normally it is not possible to identify cases at the start of the preclinical phase and to relate sensitivity to this point. In an unscreened population, however, clinical diagnosis indicates the *end* of the preclinical phase. Therefore, the sensitivity function can be thought of as the average probability of detection of cases that are a given amount of time away from clinical diagnosis. In other words, the sensitivity function gives the sensitivity of the test in relation to the *potential* lead time. The degree of manifestation tested for will vary among cases with a given potential lead time. As a result, some cases will be highly detectable, others moderately so, and some cases will be only slightly detectable or entirely undetectable. Like the detectability of an individual case, the level of the sensitivity function increases as the

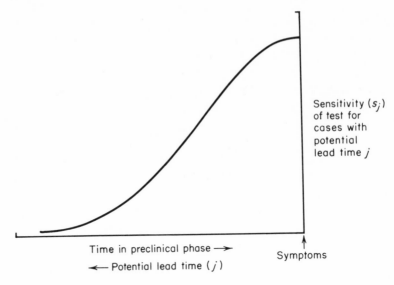

Figure 3-5. Illustration of a sensitivity function.

Source: Adapted from Eddy (1980).

time of diagnosis approaches; a sensitivity function might have the appearance shown in Figure 3-5. The quantity j is the interval between the time of screening and the time that clinical diagnosis would occur if the disease were not detected; that is, j is the potential lead time. For the cases that are detected, j also is the actual lead time. The quantity s_j is the sensitivity of the screening test for cases that have a potential lead time of j. Suppose that, at the time of testing, there are k_j preclinical cases with time between j and $j + \Delta t$ until diagnosis as a result of symptoms. The sensitivity of the test to detect such cases (s_j) is the number of cases detected ($c_j = l_j - l_{j+\Delta t}$) divided by the total available (k_j), or $s_j = c_j/k_j$. The sensitivity function of the test is, then, the series of sensitivities that corresponds to a series of potential lead times denoted by j. As stated at the beginning of this chapter, the sensitivity of a procedure is generally taken to be its ability to detect a given amount of a substance. The sensitivity function of a screening test describes its ability to detect a given amount of disease as measured by its potential lead time.

As with the overall sensitivity, the value of the sensitivity function c_j/k_j for a given potential lead time j often cannot be estimated in practice because the true number of preclinical cases k_j cannot be determined. On the other hand, c_j is the observable number of *detected* preclinical cases that appear in the lead-time distribution. Therefore, the sensitivity functions of two or more tests (including diagnostic tests) can be compared in *relative* terms by use of lead-time distributions generated by the tests. Suppose that two tests, A and B, are applied to identical groups of people. The numbers of cases that gain a lead time of i to $i + \Delta t$ are c_j^A and c_j^B, respectively. Since the two groups are equivalent except for the test applied, it can be assumed that the numbers of cases with potential lead time of j to $j + \Delta t$ are identical, that is, $k_j^A = k_j^B$. Thus, the sensitivity of test A in detecting cases $j = i$ time units before clinical diagnosis, relative to the corresponding sensitivity of test B, is equal to the ratio of the respective numbers of detected cases with lead time of i to $i + \Delta t$

$$\frac{s_j^A}{s_j^B} = \frac{c_i^A / k_j^A}{c_i^B / k_j^B} = \frac{c_i^A}{c_i^B} \tag{3-6}$$

This expression is given primarily for background rather than practical application; complete lead-time distributions are not likely to be used very often in evaluating test sensitivity. A long period of observation, perhaps several years, may be required to determine a lead-time distribution; information on sensitivity usually is needed more rapidly. Furthermore, lead-time distributions may have substantial statistical uncertainty associated with them. Even though screening programs often involve thousands of subjects, the numbers of cases from which lead-time distributions are estimated usually are rather small. In the HIP study, for example, there were only 132 screen-detected cases. Finally, the lead-time distributions to be compared would have to be determined on separate populations. If one group is screened with both tests, separate lead-time distributions for each test cannot be determined since it is not possible to ascertain when, or whether, a given case, detected as positive by one test, would have been detected by the other.

Nonetheless, the relative sensitivity function given by expression (3-6) is helpful for interpreting other measures of sensitivity. If a test is applied to a population, the total number of detected cases, C_{0s}, is equal to the sum of the numbers of cases with lead time in the various intervals. That is,

$$C_{0s} = \Sigma c_i = \Sigma s_j k_j$$

If two tests (A and B) are applied to identical populations or applied independently to the same population, so that the numbers of preclinical cases available for detection are equal, then

$$C_{0s}^A = \Sigma s_j^A k_j \quad \text{and} \quad C_{0s}^B = \Sigma s_j^B k_j$$

The ratio C_{0s}^A / C_{0s}^B is the ratio of the prevalence of preclinical disease detected by test A to the prevalence detected by test B. If the relative sensitivity function of the tests is constant with the amount of potential lead time, then C_{0s}^A/C_{0s}^B is equal to the constant relative sensitivity. Even if the individual relative sensitivities are not constant, the ratio of cases detected with one test to cases detected with the other is equivalent to the ratio of the sensitivities of the two tests as defined in the customary manner, since the number positive to a diagnostic test would be the same for each screening test:

$$\frac{C_{0s}^A}{C_{0s}^B} = \frac{\dfrac{C_{0s}^A}{\text{Number positive to diagnostic test}}}{\dfrac{C_{0s}^B}{\text{Number positive to diagnostic test}}} = \frac{s_{.}^A}{s_{.}^B}$$

If test B is a diagnostic test, then

$$s_{.}^B = \frac{\text{Number positive to diagnostic test}}{\text{Number positive to diagnostic test}} = 1$$

and $s_{.}^A/s_{.}^B = s_{.}^A$ is the sensitivity of test A as usually defined.

Another measure of sensitivity discussed was the ratio of the number of cases detected to that number plus the number diagnosed in a given follow-up interval. As indicated, the value obtained for this measure of sensitivity is related to the length of the follow-up interval selected. However, the ratio of two program sensitivities (the proportion of cases found by screening among all cases diagnosed during a screening program = C_{0s}/C_{Tm}) is identical to C_{0s}^A/C_{0s}^B since the denominators of the two estimates would be the same.

Sensitivity also may be described as the ratio of the number of cases detected by a particular test to the number detected by all tests in use. Thus, the sensitivity of test A would be estimated as

$$\frac{C_{0s}^A}{C_{0s}^A + C_{0s}^B + C_{0s}^C + \cdots}$$

This is the measure on page 47 in comparing the sensitivities of mammography, thermography, and physical examination in screening for breast cancer. This estimate of the sensitivity of a test decreases with the total number of tests in use, but the ratio of sensitivities determined in this way is again C_{0s}^A/C_{0s}^B regardless of the number of tests used.

Since the lead-time distribution generated by a test depends on prevailing medical care and awareness, the apparent sensitivity characteristics of a test are best regarded as specific to the circumstances in which they are evaluated. Furthermore, the sensitivity will appear relatively high at the

Table 3–4. Percentages of Screen-detected Cases of Breast Cancer in the HIP Study That Were Detected by Physical Examination and by Mammography

Type of examination	Age at detection			
	40–49	50–59	60+	All ages
Physical exam only	61%	41%	37%	45%
Mammography only	19	41	31	33
Physical exam and mammography	19	18	31	22

Source: Shapiro et al (1988).

first screen in a continuing program, because prevalent preclinical cases at the time of the first screen tend to be relatively advanced and easy to detect, compared to cases tested at later screens (Chamberlain et al, 1984).

The apparent sensitivity of a test may depend on various characteristics of the people screened. In the HIP study, for example, mammography was more sensitive (relative to physical examination) in women 50 years of age or older than it was in younger women (Table 3–4). The radiologic characteristics of breast tissue change with age and these changes are likely to affect the probability that a tumor is observed on a mammogram. Radiologic features of the breast also depend on body fatness (Brisson et al, 1982b, 1984), so the sensitivity of mammography also may be related to obesity.

Variations in test sensitivity for such reasons will cause differences in lead-time distributions among subsets of participants in a screening program, and these differences could affect respective reductions of morbidity or mortality. The relation of the lead-time distribution to age can be assessed by classifying program participants according to age at screening and then deriving an estimate of the distribution for each age group. The lead time in detection of tumors of a specific site might also vary according to histologic characteristics of the tumor. For example, different lead-time distributions might be obtained in cytologic screening for high-grade (more malignant) *v* low-grade (less malignant) tumors of the bladder, since high-grade tumors seem to be detected more readily (Farrow, 1979). To derive lead-time distributions for tumors of different histologic types, these should be thought of as distinct diseases. Derivation of the distribution for each type would involve only the dates of diagnosis of that type in the screened and comparison groups. Unfortunately, the usefulness of data on lead time in subgroups of a screened population is likely to be limited by the relatively small number of cases available in most screening programs. Obviously, the lead time cannot be evaluated in relation to a characteristic that is changed by early detection. For example, it would be meaningless to assess the lead time of low-stage breast cancer. The screening program itself creates low-stage cases; the stage is a reflection of the lead time.

MATHEMATICAL MODELS IN ESTIMATING LEAD TIME

Some estimates of the amount of lead time gained by screening have been derived by use of mathematical models (Albert et al, 1978a,b; Hutchison and Shapiro, 1968; Prorok, 1976a,b; Walter and Day, 1983; Zelen and Feinleib, 1969). In such models, the distribution of the duration of pre-clinical disease, which implies the lead-time distribution, typically is assumed to have a particular shape. Estimates of average lead time may be obtained from models by use of data as simple as the detected prevalence of the disease in screened persons and the incidence rate in unscreened persons.

The models used to estimate lead time typically require an assumption regarding the course of detectability during the preclinical phase, that is, the sensitivity function. A simple assumption that has frequently been made is that the preclinical phase of the disease screened for has two segments: the time during which the disease is essentially undetectable by the test to be used (sensitivity = 0), and the time during which the disease would be detected by the test if it were applied (sensitivity = 100%.) The second segment might be called the uniformly detectable preclinical phase (UDPP). As with the preclinical phase in general, the UDPP refers to the entire period that would exist *without* screening. In other words, detection does not change the length of the UDPP.

A model also may involve the assumption that the disease in the screened population is in a steady state. If this condition holds, the UDPP of the disease has a constant incidence rate (I_p) and a constant distribution of duration (d_p). No real population is truly in a steady state, although steady-state conditions are approximated reasonably well in many situations. If a previously unscreened population has been screened recently, it is not in a steady state, since the distribution of the duration of preclinical disease that remains undiagnosed after screening is changing toward the pattern that existed before. With the passage of time, and no further screening, the prescreening distribution is restored and maintained.

In a steady-state population, the average duration of the UDPP, $\bar{d}_p$, is equal to its prevalence P divided by its incidence rate I_p (Freeman and Hutchison, 1980).

$$\bar{d}_p = \frac{P}{I_p} \tag{3-7}$$

If such a population is screened, the prevalence of detectable preclinical disease P is given by the number of cases detected divided by the number screened. Usually, the incidence rate of detectable preclinical disease I_p is not known. If the UDPP does not tend to be too long, however, I_p may be approximated by I_c, the incidence rate of clinical disease (Morrison, 1979a). Then,

$$\overline{d}_p \doteq \frac{P}{I_c} \tag{3-8}$$

The validity of expressions (3–7) and (3–8) depends on the validity of the assumptions on which the expressions are based. The size and direction of any error would depend on the specific way in which the conditions are violated. Suppose, for example, that the average duration of the UDPP is long compared to the induction period of preclinical disease. Then the incidence rate of clinical disease (I_c) will be substantially less than the incidence rate of preclinical disease (I_p). One source of such a difference would be the existence of pseudodisease. The consequence of this error would be that the estimate of the average duration of the UDPP from (3–8) would be too long in relation to disease that ultimately would become clinical without screening. Departure from steady-state conditions also will lead to error. If the incidence rate of preclinical disease were increasing rapidly, but the distribution of the length of the UDPP did not change, the observed prevalence would be lower than the ultimate steady-state prevalence. Therefore, the estimated duration of the UDPP would be too low.

A case detected by a one-time screening program in a steady-state population would, on the average, be detected midway through the UDPP. Therefore, the average lead time experienced by screen-detected cases would be one-half the average duration of the UDPP of those screen-detected cases. If all cases, whether screen-detected or not, have the same length detectable preclinical phase, then the average lead time would be

$$\overline{L} = \tfrac{1}{2}\,\overline{d}_p \doteq \tfrac{1}{2}\frac{P}{I_c} \tag{3-9}$$

In general, however, the duration of the UDPP will vary. If so, cases detected by screening would be expected to have longer UDPPs than would cases that are not detected, since the probability of detection is in proportion to the duration of the UDPP. This relation is illustrated in Figure 3–6 (Feinleib and Zelen, 1969). One-half of the detectable preclinical cases are shown to have a UDPP of four years' duration, and one-half have a UDPP of one year's duration. If screening is done, four long cases are detected for each short one. The average duration of the UDPP of all detectable preclinical cases is 2.5 years, but the average duration of the

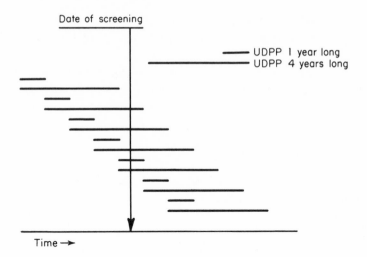

Mean duration of UDPP of all cases = $\dfrac{4+1}{2}$ = 2.5 years

Mean duration of UDPP of screen-detected cases = $\dfrac{4(4)+1}{5}$ = 3.4 years

Figure 3–6. Illustration of the relationship between the mean duration of the uniformly detectable preclinical phase (UDPP) detection by screening.

Source: Feinleib and Zelen (1969).

UDPP of cases actually detected is 3.4 years. Thus, the average lead time is ½ × 3.4 years = 1.7 years, which is greater than 1.25 years, one-half the duration of the UDPP of all cases. Variation in the length of the UDPP could even lead to the paradox that cases discovered in a one-time screening program have a greater average lead time than that of cases discovered in a program of very frequent screening that maximizes the earliness of detection (Hutchison and Shapiro, 1968). If one-tenth of all cases have a UDPP 9 years long, and nine-tenths have a UDPP of 1 year, equal numbers of cases of each length would be detected in a one-time program, and the mean lead time would be (4.5 years + 0.5 year)/2 = 2.5 years. On the other hand, if screening were so frequent that every case is discovered virtually at the start of the UDPP, the mean lead time would be

$$\frac{(9 \text{ years} \times 1) + (1 \text{ year} \times 9)}{10} = 1.8 \text{ years}$$

The average lead time per detected case is reduced by frequent screening because a much higher proportion of cases with short UDPPs are detected by frequent than by infrequent screening. The total lead time gained by all detected cases will, of course, increase with the frequency of screening, as will the lead time that a given case gains.

Hutchison and Shapiro (1968) showed that the mean lead time of cases detected by a screening examination applied once to a steady-state population is

$$\overline{L} = \tfrac{1}{2}\left(\overline{d}_p + \frac{V_p}{\overline{d}_p}\right) \tag{3-10}$$

where V_p is the variance of the distribution of duration of the UDPP of all cases, whether screen-detected or not. If all cases have the same length UDPP, the variance is zero and expression (3–10) reduces to expression (3–9). However, if the length of the UDPP does vary, the average lead time would be greater than that derived by using expression (3–9) as a result of the positive value of V_p. Thus, expression (3–10) is a general form of expression (3–9), which allows for the amount of variation in the length of the UDPP.

Hutchison and Shapiro used expression (3–10) to estimate the average lead time gained at the first and subsequent screenings in the HIP study. In that study, 2.7 cases of breast cancer were discovered per 1,000 women screened at the initial examination. The incidence rate I_p of preclinical breast cancer was estimated from I_c, the incidence rate of clinical breast cancer in the control group, as 1.6 per 1,000 person-years (PY). Thus, the mean duration of the UDPP was estimated as

$$\overline{d}_p \doteq \frac{P}{I_c} = \frac{2.7 \text{ per } 1,000}{1.6 \text{ per } 1,000 \text{ PY}} = 1.7 \text{ years}$$

If the duration of the UDPP were constant (ie, $V_p = 0$), the mean lead time generated by the initial screening examination would be

$$\overline{L} = \tfrac{1}{2}\,\overline{d}_p = \tfrac{1}{2} \times 1.7 \text{ years} = 10 \text{ months}$$

Assuming that the duration of the UDPP varies ($V_p > 0$), the value of $\overline{L}$ would be greater than 10 months. Hutchison and Shapiro obtained estimates of $\overline{L}$ with V_p's corresponding to various hypothetical distributions of the duration of the UDPP. The mean lead time would be 1.6 years if the distribution were a negative exponential.

Compared to breast cancer, the detectable phase of preclinical cervical cancer tends to be much longer. Data on age at diagnosis of screen-detected v routinely diagnosed cases suggest an average duration of as much as three decades (Task Force, 1976). Zelen and Feinleib (1969) described a way to use information on age at diagnosis to estimate mean lead time without the necessity of knowing or assuming the nature of the distribution of duration of the UDPP. Suppose that this distribution is not related to age. If there are no deaths from other diseases, the mean age at which cases come to medical attention in an unscreened population, $\overline{A}_{I_c}$, is equal to the mean age at which the UDPP develops, $\overline{A}_{I_p}$, plus the mean duration of the UDPP, $\overline{d}_p$.

$$\overline{A}_{I_c} = \overline{A}_{I_p} + \overline{d}_p$$

Furthermore, the mean age at which screen-detected disease is diagnosed, $\overline{A}_p$, is equal to $\overline{A}_{I_p}$ plus one-half the mean duration of the UDPP of the cases detected, $\frac{1}{2}\overline{d}_{ps}$, which is the mean lead time.

$$\overline{A}_p = \overline{A}_{I_p} + \frac{1}{2}\,\overline{d}_{ps}$$

The difference in mean ages at diagnosis of screen-detected and routinely diagnosed disease is then

$$\overline{A}_{I_c} - \overline{A}_p = \overline{d}_p - \frac{1}{2}\,\overline{d}_{ps}$$

Therefore, the mean lead time is

$$\overline{L} = \frac{1}{2}\,\overline{d}_{ps} = \overline{d}_p + \overline{A}_p - \overline{A}_{I_c} \qquad (3\text{--}11)$$

As before, $\overline{d}_p$ can be estimated from expression (3–8) so that the mean lead time can be calculated.

This method of estimating mean lead time has two limitations in addition to the assumptions regarding the UDPP and steady-state conditions. First, there is no particular reason to believe that the distribution of duration of the UDPP is constant with age. The length of the clinical phase of many diseases varies with age and it is likely that the preclinical phase does the same. Such variation could lead to either positive or negative bias in expression (3–11). Second, the estimation procedure is based on what the average age at diagnosis would be if there were no deaths from other diseases. Since deaths do occur from other diseases, these averages must be derived from age-specific incidence rates of the target disease. The rates of many diseases rise with age, and rates are not available for ages above 80 or so, because few people live much past that age. Thus, for many diseases, the set of age-specific rates to be averaged is truncated (Albert et al, 1978a). As a consequence of truncation, the observed values of $\overline{A}_{I_c}$ and $\overline{A}_p$ may be too close. This leads to a positive bias in the estimate of mean lead time if $\overline{A}_{I_c}$ is greater than $\overline{A}_p$ and a negative bias if $\overline{A}_{I_c}$ is less than $\overline{A}_p$.

RELATION OF THE LEAD-TIME DISTRIBUTION TO THE DISTRIBUTION OF DURATION OF PRECLINICAL DISEASE: Through measurements of the frequency of diagnosed disease, the lead-time distribution can be directly observed in the course of a screening program. However, the distribution of the duration of the preclinical phase (the source of the lead time) is a more fundamental concept than the lead time for describing the natural history of a disease since the lead time only exists if screening is done. If the distribution of the duration of the preclinical phase were available, the rate at which pre-clinical disease becomes clinical could be estimated: In a steady state, the average duration of preclinical disease (assuming no removal for other causes) is the inverse of the rate of transition from preclinical to clinical, just as the life expectancy is the inverse of the mortality rate from all causes (Morrison, 1979a).

Unfortunately, the distribution of the length of the preclinical phase is very difficult to evaluate. For one thing, the total length of the preclinical phase cannot be determined unless a perfect test is available. Therefore, it is necessary to restrict attention to preclinical disease that is detectable by the test in use. Most approaches to estimating the duration of the detectable preclinical phase are based on the same types of models that are used to estimate mean lead time. These models assume the existence of a UDPP and provide estimates of the average, but not the distribution, of its length. The observed lead-time distribution (expression (3–2)) can be used to suggest the shape of the distribution of the length of the UDPP (J. Brisson, written communication, 1980[2]). However, such an estimate would only be useful if very large amounts of data were available, since the statistical uncertainty in the estimated lead-time distribution is further increased when this distribution is used to estimate yet another distribution.

Walter and Day (1983) developed models of the relation between the distribution of the duration of the detectable preclinical phase of a disease and the sensitivity of a test to the detected prevalence at each screening examination in a series and the incidence of symptomatic disease, by time, among persons who test negative at each of the screens. They assumed that the sensitivity of the test is constant during the detectable preclinical phase and that the sensitivity is constant from case to case, and from one screen to the next.

Walter and Day derived simultaneous estimates of the parameters of the distribution of the duration of preclinical disease and the sensitivity of screening by use of prevalence and incidence data from the HIP study. The method they used depends on knowledge of the incidence of clinical illness among unscreened persons. The incidence may be derived as an additional estimate based on data from screened persons or it may be fur-nished from an external source (the controls in the HIP study). Higher precision is obtained by use of external incidence data since the need to estimate it in the model is avoided.

Of the distributions that Walter and Day investigated, the negative expo-nential fit the data best. With this distribution they estimated the mean duration of detectable preclinical disease as 1.7 years. If the distribution of the duration of preclinical disease is actually negative exponential, the mean duration of preclinical disease and the mean lead time would be the same.

The negative exponential distribution may provide a satisfactory description of the progression of preclinical disease in some bodies of data. This distribution implies, however, that the rate of transition to clinical illness does not depend on the time spent in the preclinical phase. This condition is probably not met for individual cases. It seems likely that the risk of clinical illness increases with time in the preclinical phase. Thus, predictions based on the negative exponential assumption should be used with caution.

Walter and Day treat the sensitivity of testing as conceptually distinct from the distribution of the duration of the preclinical phase. If, however, it is not possible to determine the prevalence of preclinical disease independently of screening, their model is effectively based on a one-step sensitivity function without explicit consideration of the length of the preclinical phase. The sensitivity would be zero for an initial period that is of indeterminate length, and the sensitivity would then jump to a constant value which is greater than zero. Estimates would be obtained of the sensitivity after the step and of the distribution of its length, which would be the same as the distribution of the duration of detectable preclinical disease.

Walter and Day point out that their model imposes a negative correlation between the mean duration of preclinical disease and the sensitivity, because an increase in one must be compensated by a decrease in the other to account for a given detected prevalence. Furthermore, the assumption that the sensitivity is constant during the detectable preclinical phase is implausible. It is more likely that detectability increases as the end of the preclinical phase approaches (Figure 3–5). If such a relation were built into the model, the correlation between the sensitivity and the duration of preclinical disease would increase (Day and Walter, 1984). Day and Walter suggest that a high correlation of the two is undesirable and a reason not to include increasing detectability in the model. Because of the equivalence of their model to a model based on a one-step sensitivity function, however, there is nothing to lose, and possibly something to gain, by a more realistic description of the relation between the progression of disease and its detectability.

To the extent that models of preclinical disease, or lead time, and sensitivity conform to the biology of disease progression and detection, they are useful in describing and understanding those processes. The estimates from such models may be used to provide guidance as to screening schedules or age groups to be screened. Such estimates may also provide early indications of the effectiveness of new or modified methods of screening in comparison to methods that have already been evaluated (Walter and Day, 1983; Day and Walter, 1984). At present, however, there is little understanding of the relation between the lead-time distribution achieved by screening and the subsequent reduction in mortality. Individual lead times longer than those necessary for effective treatment are not beneficial and may be harmful. Data on screening for breast cancer or cervical cancer suggest that increasingly early detection may not offer commensurate benefits.

NOTES

[1]A lead-time distribution can be derived from differences between screened and unscreened groups in the prevalent numbers of diagnosed cases, the cumulative numbers diagnosed, or, as mentioned on page 54, the diagnosis rates, by time after screening. Although they are obviously interrelated, these approaches are not entirely equivalent. The prevalent numbers (with correction for the effect of treatment) give the lead times actually experienced. As time passes, deaths from other causes reduce the prevalent number of screen-detected cases that would otherwise continue to experience lead time. This reduction does not affect lead times determined from either the cumulative numbers of diagnosed cases or the incidence rates, since these approaches do not involve continuing observation of cases after diagnosis. In contrast to lead-time distributions derived from either prevalent or cumulative numbers, a distribution derived from incidence rates does not reflect the second type of pseudodisease described on page 24 (screen-detected cases that would progress but die of another cause before symptoms develop) since incidence rates intrinsically compensate for deaths from other (independent) causes.

[2]If the length of the UDPP has a constant value T, the probability that the lead time would exceed t (for t in the interval from 0 to T) is $(T - t)/T$. Since the longest *observed* value of the lead time is T_m, the lead time would have a uniform distribution with values ranging from 0 to approximately T_m. Now suppose that the length of the UDPP varies. Let the probability that the length takes a value in the interval from T to $T + \Delta t$ (for T in the interval from 0 to $T_m - \Delta t$) be P_T. Then, the probability that the lead time would take some value $\geq t$ is

$$\sum_{T=t}^{T_m - \Delta t} \frac{T - t}{T} P_T$$

Since this probability of a lead time $\geq t$ is also estimated as l_t/C_{0s},

$$\frac{l_t}{C_{0s}} = \sum_{T=t}^{T_m - \Delta t} \frac{T - t}{T} P_T \tag{3–12}$$

For a lead time in the interval $T_m - \Delta t$ to T_m,

$$P_{T_m} - \Delta t = \frac{l_{T_m} - \Delta t}{C_{0s}}$$

This value can be substituted in expression (3–12), which can be solved for $P_{T_m} - 2\Delta t$, etc.

4 Assessing the Value of Early Treatment: Experimental Studies

The long-term benefit to be derived from screening is the reduction of morbidity or mortality. This chapter and chapter 5 are concerned with methods of assessing the extent of this reduction.

BACKGROUND

Epidemiology deals broadly with the evaluation of exposure-disease relationships. *Exposures* include causal agents such as cigarette smoke or bacteria, preventive measures such as dietary improvement or immunization, therapies for symptomatic disease, and programs for the detection and treatment of asymptomatic disease. Disease occurrence may be marked by an initial diagnosis, evidence of recurrence or progression, or death from the disease.

A person's total experience with an exposure depends on the characteristics of each encounter, and their number and spacing. A given encounter may be described in terms of dose, eg, the amount of radiation delivered or the quantity of a vaccine injected, or in terms of technical features, such as the way in which an examination or operation is done. The number and spacing of exposures can be summarized by the age at which exposure begins, the rate at which encounters occur, and any changes in this rate with time. From this perspective, the simplest type of exposure is that which occurs only once—a *point exposure*. Radiation from an atomic bomb blast is a well-known example. A single immunization, or a single screening examination (followed by treatment of the cases detected), are additional examples. In describing a point exposure, the age at the encounter must be specified and, if appropriate, the dose or technique, but issues of the rate or duration of exposure are not applicable.

Recurrent exposures obviously are more difficult to characterize. Consider exposure to cigarette smoke. Exposure occurs frequently but irregularly during waking hours, and ceases during sleep. The number of cigarettes smoked per day varies from smoker to smoker. For a given smoker, this number varies from day to day, and the daily number may change abruptly or gradually over the years. A smoker may or may not continue to smoke throughout life. Someone who quits may later resume the habit at the same or a different average intensity as before.

In smokers, encounters with cigarettes typically occur many times a day, and the number of cigarettes or packs smoked per day is a useful measure of the rate of exposure. If smoking, once begun, is continued at a roughly constant rate, then smoking exposure can be summarized well by the age at which it began and the average daily rate. If there are substantial changes in this rate with time, then a good summary would incorporate them. The exposure could be described by a function of intensity according to age; the intensity would be zero during periods of discontinuation.

Similar comments apply to the temporal characterization of screening. Typically, however, screening is repeated at intervals of a year or more, rather than many times a day as smoking is. Therefore, descriptions of screening schedules usually refer to periods at least several years long.

Sometimes an exposure is expressed cumulatively. For example, the risk of bladder cancer has been related to the cumulative number of cigarettes smoked (Howe et al, 1980). The cumulative exposure depends, however, on the average exposure rate and the length of the period of exposure; the same cumulative exposure may be the result of a long period of exposure at a low rate, or a short intensive exposure. Unless information to the contrary is available, it should be assumed that the effect of an exposure depends on both its rate and its duration. The effect of two screening examinations could differ markedly depending on whether they were given a day or two years apart. Thus, it may be misleading to use cumulative measures to summarize an exposure. Duration and intensity should be investigated separately.

Exposure to a causal, preventive, or therapeutic agent leads to changes in the subsequent rate of disease events. The changes may be abrupt, as in an acute outbreak due to bacterial infection: The rate rises and then returns to its preepidemic level within the span of a few days or weeks. On the other hand, the changes may be slow: The effect of ionizing radiation on the rate of breast cancer takes at least 10 years to become apparent, and it is not yet known when, or even if, a subsequent decrease occurs (Boice et al, 1991).

Evaluation of an exposure-disease relationship is done by means of comparisons of disease rates among groups defined according to exposure pattern. The disease experience of people with a given exposure pattern is often summarized by a single figure such as an average rate. The full description of an exposure-disease relationship, however, gives changes in the disease rate according to time beginning with entry into each exposure category and continuing until the exposure no longer has an effect on the rate.

In the evaluation of screening, the approach that has been used most frequently is the comparison of survival or cumulative case fatality between screen-detected cases and cases not detected by screening. This approach does not meet a basic criterion of validity—that the comparison not be expected to show a difference when, in truth, none exists. The survival experience of a group of screen-detected cases may depend in large part on diagnostic effects of screening—lead time and prognostic selection—and, therefore, differ from the survival experience of routinely diagnosed cases even if early treatment does not postpone death. This problem is discussed at length in chapter 6.

There are two general types of comparisons of morbidity or mortality that avoid biases from the diagnostic effects of screening. First, morbidity or mortality may be compared between initially nondiseased groups defined according to screening exposure. This is the method that is used most often, and it will be described in detail.

Second, subjects with asymptomatic disease may be identified by screening. Assuming that it is not considered imperative to treat these subjects, rates of the outcome events may be compared between groups that are, and that are not, treated while asymptomatic. The effects of treating screen-detected hypertension and hyperlipidemia have been investigated in this way (chapter 10). This method has the advantage of relative simplicity. Once the diseased subjects are identified, all subsequent effort is focused on them. The large number of subjects initially screened negative, and additional unscreened subjects, are not kept under surveillance as they would be in the first method.

The simplicity of the second method, however, is offset by important disadvantages. Because of the lack of surveillance of persons screened negative and of unscreened persons, it is not possible to evaluate directly the proportion of serious morbidity or mortality from the disease that is prevented by screening and early treatment. Furthermore, the method does not provide information on the lead time or sensitivity of screening, information that may be helpful in formulating a screening policy. In general, therefore, this method should not be used if positive results from a study are likely to lead to recommendations for population screening.

Whichever method is used, the specific outcome events to be assessed must be defined carefully. In a study of screening, a new diagnosis of the disease of interest usually is an inappropriate outcome, since screening itself brings about early diagnosis. Consequently, a screened population would have a higher rate of initial diagnosis than an otherwise comparable unscreened population would. Through the first four years of observation in the HIP study, 250 cases of breast cancer were identified in the study group compared to 219 in the control group (Table 3–3). This difference subsequently narrowed, but it presumably would have been maintained if screening had continued. Thus, the measured rate of diagnosis was raised about 14% by screening. Generally, a screened population would have an elevated rate of any medical event related to the disease of interest that occurs during the lead-time interval. This difference is in the opposite direction to a beneficial effect of early treatment on mortality. It also is inappropriate to attempt to evaluate screening programs by comparing the extent or severity of disease at the time of diagnosis between screen-detected v routinely diagnosed cases. Any differences observed might well reflect only lead time, not later health status.

If early treatment is beneficial, it reduces morbidity or mortality after the time that diagnosis would occur if there is no screening, that is, after the lead-time interval. Therefore, a study should assess late, rather than early, manifestations of the disease process. Death from the disease obviously meets this criterion, and mortality is generally viewed as the most readily interpretable outcome in studies of the efficacy of screening (Prorok et al, 1981). The following discussion focuses on death from the disease as the outcome event in a screening program. As pointed out in chapter 1, it must be assumed that cause-of-death certification does not depend on whether or not a case is screen-detected. If it does, interpretation of the apparent value of a screening program, even in the context of an experimental trial, could be quite uncertain.

Death is not, however, the only appropriate outcome in the evaluation of screening. At times, death may even be an inappropriate measure. The occurrence of blindness would be the best outcome event to use in a study of the value of screening for glaucoma. Death rates would provide little, if any, information on the problem. Even when death would be the most suitable outcome in principle, there are certain practical circumstances, especially in case-control studies, when other outcomes may be useful. In general, screened and unscreened groups can appropriately be compared on the basis of rates of development of manifestations of advanced symptomatic illness. From the point of view of study design and analysis, such outcomes can be regarded as death would be.

As with any exposure-disease relationship, the effects of early treatment may be evaluated by either experimental or nonexperimental means. The experimental approach is described in this chapter; the nonexperimental approach is described in chapter 5.

Experimental methods have been discussed extensively. Some general references are Hennekins and Buring (1987), Hutchison (1981), Peto et al (1976, 1977), and Weiss (1986).

An experimental or intervention study is a follow-up study in which the subjects are *assigned*, usually at random, to the exposures whose effects are being compared. In a valid experimental study with a nonrandom method of assignment, the subjects behave *as if* they have been allocated at random. Follow-up of subjects should begin at entry into the study, and entry should be defined in a way that is the same for each exposure category. This goal is often achieved by treating the time of assignment as the time of entry. The start of exposure is also a suitable entry point as long as the intervals from assignment to exposure are the same among the groups compared. If, however, the time of entry is taken as the completion of exposure, the composition and even the disease experience of the groups may differ if the respective exposures have different durations or different short-term complications.

In experimental studies, estimates of the effects of the exposures are usually derived from the cumulative proportions of disease events assessed at one or more intervals after the start of observation. Random allocation tends to distribute follow-up intervals uniformly among the groups compared. As a result, the observed proportions accurately reflect differences in rates among the groups. Moreover, these proportions are very simple statistics to calculate, as are the corresponding confidence intervals and significance tests (Rothman, 1986, 168–174). Curves of observed rates according to time also may be derived from experimental data.

THE HIP STUDY

This study is a landmark because of its methods, its results, and the detail given in published analyses (Shapiro et al, 1988). It is discussed at length here because it illustrates many important aspects of the evaluation and use of screening in disease control. The impetus for the HIP study came from work done in the early 1960s. Gershon-Cohen et al (1961) showed that mammography could detect breast tumors that were not palpable, and Egan (1962) showed that mammographic findings could often distinguish malignant neoplasia from benign conditions. Also, it was apparent that breast cancer detected by mammography tended to be localized (Stevens and Weigen, 1966; Witten and Thurber, 1964). Although it was suspected that the prognosis of patients with early breast cancer was good, the value of early detection in reducing the mortality rate from breast cancer was uncertain. A pilot study done by the HIP, and a study of the reliability of mammography (Clark et al, 1965), supported the feasibility of a large-scale experiment.

The HIP is a comprehensive, prepaid medical insurance plan. Care is provided by a number of participating group practices. There were 62,000 women aged 40 to 64 years (members of HIP for at least one year) who were identified for study. These women were stratified by age, family size, and the type of employment on which HIP membership was based. Then, the women were assigned alternatively, based on identification number, to the study (screened) group or the control (usual care) group. Since the assignment of the identification number was not related to any personal characteristics, the method of allocation to study and control groups was effectively random. Assuming that screening is associated with a 20% reduction in cumulative mortality and that two-thirds of the women invited to participate would actually do so, the study size of about 60,000— 30,000 in each group—would provide a 50% chance of observing a difference between study and control groups in the number of deaths from breast cancer over five years of observation that would be statistically significant with $P \leq .1$ (Shapiro et al, 1968).

Each woman in the study group was invited to have a screening examination for breast cancer, and each woman who had one (without cancer being found) was asked to appear for three annual follow-up examinations. Members of the control group were not screened, but were eligible for all HIP benefits that included, if desired, general physical examinations. The date on which a woman in the study group was scheduled for her initial screening examination was considered her entry date, and the corresponding member of the control group was assigned the same date for use in follow-up and analysis.

The screening examination consisted of cephalocaudad and lateral x-rays of each breast, and a physical examination of the breasts done by a physician, usually a surgeon. Every screened woman had both types of examination. The x-ray and physical findings were assessed and recorded independently. Although the HIP study was prompted by the development of mammography, physical examination was included as part of the screening procedure because it was known that some tumors were palpable but not visible on x-ray. Since the two types of screening were done separately, it was possible to determine which type of test was responsible for the detection of each case.

Recommendations for biopsy were made after consideration of both clinical and x-ray findings, and positive biopsies were followed by treatment. The most frequently used surgical procedure was radical mastectomy. Although surgical treatment did not follow a specific protocol, women in the two assigned groups appeared to have been treated equivalently. Surveillance of study and control groups was maintained in order to identify cases of breast cancer not detected by screening and to identify deaths from any cause. Known cases of breast cancer were followed up intensively.

The initial round of screening was carried out in the period 1963 to 1966. Sixty-five percent of the women in the study group had the initial examination. Of the women who responded to the request for the initial examination, 80% had the first reexamination, 73% the second reexamination, and 69% the third. Thirty-nine percent of the 31,000 women in the study group had all four examinations.

During the first five years of observation, 304 breast cancers were diagnosed in the study group, and 298 in the control group. Of the cases in the study group, 132 were detected by screening, 55 at the first examination. Those not detected by screening were either interval cases among screened women, or cases diagnosed among members of the study group who refused to participate in the screening program.

Of the total of 132 breast cancers detected by screening, 22% were detected by both physical examination and mammography, 33% were detected only by mammography, and 45% were detected only by physical examination. The proportion of cases detected by each method varied substantially with age at the time of detection; mammography was more important among older women, and physical examination was more important among younger women (Table 3–4).

The proportion of cases with histologic evidence of axillary lymph-node metastasis was lower for cases in the study group (32%) compared to the control group (42%). The lowest proportions of cases with metastases were observed among cases detected by mammography alone (16%) or physical examination alone (19%). Among cases detected by *both* screening methods, there was a fairly high proportion—41%—with lymph-node metastases. This finding suggests that, as would be expected, cases detected by both methods were relatively advanced, that is, they had relatively short lead times.

The effect of screening and early treatment on breast cancer mortality was assessed primarily in terms of differences in the cumulative number of breast cancer deaths between the study and control groups. The most detailed analyses were based on deaths among breast cancer cases diagnosed within five years of entry. Table 4–1 gives the interval-specific and cumulative numbers of breast cancer deaths, and the study-control differences, according to time after entry into the program. Because the study and control groups were the same size, proportional reductions in the numbers of deaths are equivalent to proportional reductions in cumulative mortality. Figure 4–1 illustrates the temporal relationship between screening activities in the study and breast cancer mortality.

Table 4–1. Annual and Cumulative Numbers of Deaths with Breast Cancer as the Underlying Cause among Cases of Breast Cancer in the HIP Study Diagnosed within Five Years of Entry, by Time

Completed year after entry	Deaths during year			Cumulative number of deaths		
	Study group	Control group	Difference	Study group	Control group	Difference
1	6	2	−4	6	2	−4
2	5	6	1	11	8	−3
3	6	11	5	17	19	2
4	7	19	12	24	38	14
5	15	25	10	39	63	24
6	16	25	9	55	88	33
7	16	18	2	71	106	35
8	13	10	−3	84	116	32
9	6	10	4	90	126	36
10	5	7	2	95	133	38

Source: Shapiro et al (1988).

Over the first three years of observation, the numbers of breast cancer deaths in the two groups were similar. During the fourth through sixth years, the annual breast cancer mortality was lower in the study group; the cumulative difference in deaths increased. After the sixth year, there appears to have been no systematic or substantial difference; annual breast cancer mortality in the two groups was similar. After seven years there were 35 fewer deaths in the study group than there were in the control group. The proportional reduction in mortality was 33%. If the subsequent study-control difference of about 35 deaths were to be maintained indefinitely—no increase in breast cancer mortality in the study group compared to the control group—it could be concluded that 27% of the 132 screen-detected cases, and about 12% of the roughly 300 cases diagnosed by any means during the first five years of the program, who otherwise would have died of breast cancer, were cured by early treatment.[1] The timing of the reduction in mortality reflects the natural history of the cases that benefited: Most or all of these cases would have died in less than six years after diagnosis. Therefore, these cases were progressing relatively quickly.

The study-control difference in breast cancer deaths was somewhat larger if cases diagnosed during additional years after entry were included. The ten-year cumulative difference was 46 deaths for cases diagnosed within six years of entry, 51 for cases within seven years, 47 for cases within eight years, 46 for cases within nine years, and 46 for cases diagnosed within 10 years of entry. The proportional reduction in breast cancer mor-

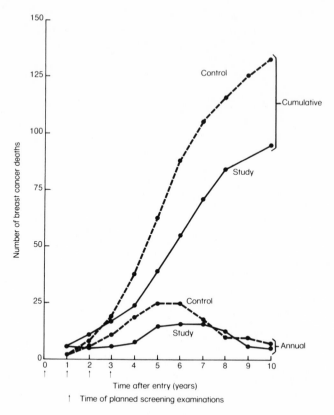

Figure 4-1. Annual and cumulative numbers of deaths from breast cancer in the HIP study.

Source: Shapiro (1977).

tality after ten years of observation is almost equal—at about 29%—for cases diagnosed within five or within seven years of entry. The proportional reduction is about 23% for cases diagnosed within ten years of entry.

The person-years of life (PYL) gained by screening depends on the ages at death in screened *v* unscreened persons. These depend directly on the underlying mortality rate from the disease of interest and the effect of screening in reducing mortality, and inversely on the mortality rate from competing causes. The PYL gained can be measured by long-term comparison of mortality in study *v* control groups. The HIP study group gained 21.0 PYL (related to breast cancer) compared to the control group after five years of observation, 188.0 PYL after ten years, and 465.5 PYL after 18 years. The PYL gained is low after five years because screening did not begin to affect breast cancer deaths until about three years after the start of the study. The long-term increase in PYL indicates that some of the cases of breast cancer that were detected and treated early may be considered to have been cured; they died much later of unrelated causes. A complete assessment, by direct observation, of PYL gained by screening would involve follow-up until all breast cancer patients diagnosed during the program have died.

In view of the basic results of the HIP study, many additional questions come to mind. For example, what are the relative contributions of each screening method to the reduction in mortality rate? Does the amount of benefit depend on the stage of the disease at detection? Does the benefit vary with age? Are different histologic types of breast cancer affected differently by early treatment?

Answers to these questions imply an analysis of mortality or case fatality in subgroups of subjects defined in various ways. However, not all such analyses are appropriate or even possible. In the HIP study, the gain from mammography cannot be separated straightforwardly from the gain because of physical examination. Each screened subject had both types of examination, and there is no way to learn what the reduction in mortality would have been if only one test or the other had been used. If only mammography had been used, then cases that were detected by physical examination alone would have been detected later by mammography or come to medical attention because of symptoms. The data do not indicate when such cases would have died, and the counterparts of these cases in the unscreened group cannot be identified for comparison. In general, an analysis gives valid results only if the groups compared are not defined on the basis of the diagnostic effects of screening. If they are, the findings may reflect, in large part, the exposure—screening—alone, rather than any decrease in mortality because of early treatment (Prorok et al, 1981). Groups defined according to the type of examination that results in detection obviously *are* determined by the diagnostic characteristics of screening, as are groups defined by age at detection or stage at detection.

Subjects in the HIP study may appropriately be divided according to their age at entry into the program, since this age in no way depends on the diagnostic outcome of screening. The mortality findings of the HIP study according to age at entry are summarized in Table 4–2. Within the first five years of the study, the study-control difference in mortality was confined to women who were at least 50 years old at entry. Subsequently, a reduction of breast cancer mortality appeared in younger women as well. The proportional decrease in deaths in the study group did not vary strongly with age. However, 48% of the women were 40 to 49 years old, 41% were 50 to 59, and 11% were 60 to 64 when the study began. Thus, the arithmetic reduction in cumulative mortality increased with age.

The screening of some women who were 40 to 49 years old at entry

Table 4–2. Cumulative Numbers of Breast Cancer Deaths among Cases of Breast Cancer in the HIP Study Diagnosed within Five Years of Entry, by Age at Entry and Time after Entry

Age at entry (years)	Time after entry					
	5 Years		10 Years		18 Years	
	Study	Control	Study	Control	Study	Control
40–49	19	20	39	51	49	65
50–59	15	33	42	61	57	74
60–64	5	10	14	21	20	24
Total	39	63	95	133	126	163

Source: Shapiro et al (1988).

continued into their fifties. It is possible that some of the benefit gained by women who were 40 to 49 at entry resulted from the early treatment of breast cancer that was detected at age 50 or greater. A reduction in breast cancer deaths in the study group was found, however, among women 40 to 44 years old at entry. These women were screened almost entirely before age 50. In short, the results of the HIP study suggest that there is a beneficial effect of screening in relatively young women, although the effect appeared later in younger than in older women.

Table 4–3 shows the PYL gained by age in the HIP study after ten years and after 18 years of observation. The values are related to the numbers of women in the study group. The age-specific PYL gained per woman reflect the underlying increases in breast cancer mortality and mortality from other causes with age, as well as the effect of early treatment. Women 50 to 59 years old at entry experienced the greatest number of PYL gained per woman. Surprisingly, perhaps, women 60 to 64 at entry gained more PYL per woman than women 40 to 49 at entry did. Thus, the proportional effect of screening in older women in relation to their higher underlying

Table 4–3. Person-years of Life Gained per Woman in the HIP Study Group, by Time after Entry and Age at Entry

Years after entry	Age at entry (years)		
	40–49	50–59	60–64
10	.00256	.01024	.00739
18	.00982	.02109	.01901

Source: Shapiro et al (1988).

mortality from breast cancer outweighed their higher mortality from competing causes. Although the number of PYL gained per woman was higher in older than younger women, the PYL gained by the affected individuals would not have been distributed similarly by age. Among young women, a relatively few cases gained many years each; among old women, many cases gained relatively few years each.

The relation of age at screening to reduction of deaths from breast cancer is discussed further in chapter 9.

Another question concerns the value of screening in different histologic types of breast cancer. As long as the histologic type does not depend on the time of diagnosis, it is valid to relate the reduction in mortality to histology. For example, the efficacy of a screening program might be assessed for ductal and for lobular carcinoma, each histologic type being considered as a separate disease. The amount by which screening reduces mortality from ductal carcinoma of the breast could be compared to the corresponding figure for lobular carcinoma.

The HIP program led to a reduction in breast cancer mortality, but compliance with the program was incomplete. As shown in chapter 5, the experience of the group that actually had at least one examination can be used to assess the value of the program, assuming full participation. However, the special strength of an experiment is the expected equality of outcomes in the original randomized groups, and analyses that are not based on these groups must be interpreted with caution. They are out of keeping with the design, and they should be treated as analyses of nonexperimental data. Compliance with an experimental protocol might well be associated with outcome aside from any effect of the exposure.

OTHER EXAMPLES

The studies described in this section illustrate additional issues in design or interpretation. Experimental studies of screening for breast cancer are summarized and discussed in chapter 9. Experimental studies of the treatment of screen-detected hypertension or hypercholesterolemia to control cardiovascular disease are presented in chapter 10.

A study of breast cancer screening being done in Canada (Miller et al, 1981a) was designed to answer certain questions that emerged from the HIP study. Two of the most important questions are these: (1) What is the value of screening relatively young women with physical examination and mammography? (2) What is the value of mammography in addition to screening by physical examination in older women? The study protocol depended, therefore, on the age of the subjects. For women aged 40 to

49 at entry, the screened group was offered a program that included five annual physical examinations and mammography, and instruction in self-examination of the breast. The control group had an initial physical examination and instruction in breast self-examination, and annual reminders to continue self-examination. Women who entered at age 50 to 59 were divided into two groups. One was offered a program of annual mammography and physical examination, as well as instruction in breast self-examination, and the other, physical examination and breast self-examination, but not mammography.

Every experimental regimen in the Canadian study included some screening. The controls in the 40- to 49-year-old group had an initial physical examination. The only difference in the two regimens offered women aged 50 to 59 was mammography, since the goal was to evaluate the additional effect of mammography in women who are screened by physical examination. Finally, all participants were instructed in breast self-examination. The effect of mammography might be small against a background of regular physical examinations as well as self-examination. Designs such as these, in which the marginal value of an additional screening procedure is studied, emphasize the fact that the amount of change in the time of diagnosis, and any resulting reduction in mortality, depends on the setting in which the screening is done.

A nonrandomized experimental study is evaluating the addition of fecal blood testing to annual sigmoidoscopy (Flehinger et al, 1986). Colorectal cancer mortality has been observed to be lower in the group offered the additional test than in the comparison group (Winawer et al, 1991). Other studies are evaluating fecal blood testing alone (Winawer et al, 1991). One of these (Kronborg et al, 1989) has also shown a beneficial effect of screening. Neither result alone is statistically significant. Follow-up is relatively short in both positive studies.

There is little evidence that the early detection and treatment of lung cancer results in reduced mortality from the disease. Brett (1968) compared two screening programs: a chest x-ray every six months for three years *v* a chest x-ray at the beginning and end of the three-year period. Subjects were drawn from men employed in a number of factories. The lung cancer mortality rate during the first three years of the study was nearly identical in both groups.

The Mayo Clinic studied lung cancer screening among male smokers (Fontana, 1985). The screened group was urged to have a chest x-ray and sputum cytology examination every four months for six years. The control group was advised to have this set of tests yearly, but was not followed up to ensure that the tests were done. There were about 4,600 men in each group. All subjects had been screened on entry and were without known lung cancer at that time.

Table 4–4. Numbers of Cases, Percentages Asymptomatic and Stage I at Diagnosis, and Survival, in the Mayo Clinic Study of Screening for Lung Cancer

	Screened	Control
Number diagnosed	167	131
Detected while asymptomatic (%)	68	30
Stage I at diagnosis (%)	40	24
Five year survival (%)	35	15
Lung cancer mortality rate[a]	2.9	2.8

Source: Fontana (1985).
[a]Deaths per 1000 PY.

In the screened group, more cases were found, and a much higher percentage was detected by screening while they were asymptomatic, compared to the control group. Furthermore, the stage at diagnosis tended to be lower, and the five-year survival much higher, for cases in the screened group. (Brett also reported more cases, and lower case-fatality, in his intensively screened group.) Thus, screening did appear to find early cases (Table 4–4). However, the numbers of cases other than stage I at diagnosis were equal in the two groups. Thus, the higher proportion of low-stage cases in the screened group may be explained by the higher number of cases diagnosed in that group. Continued follow-up will be necessary to determine whether or not the excess cases should be interpreted as pseudodisease. After an average of seven years of follow-up per subject, the lung cancer mortality rates in the two groups were virtually equal. The results of this study emphasize the hazard of predicting a screened-control difference in mortality from simple screened-control differences in stage or survival. Studies comparing the effect of adding sputum cytology tests to regular screening with chest x-rays also have been negative (Melamed et al, 1987; Mulshine et al, 1989).

As indicated in chapter 1, the idea that regular checkups might lead to reduced mortality originated at least as early as the 1920s. This idea was not carefully evaluated, however, until the 1960s and 1970s, when an experimental study of "multiphasic" screening was carried out (Dales et al, 1979; Friedman et al, 1986). Subjects were selected from among subscribers to the Kaiser Foundation Health Plan. Those eligible were 35 to 54 years old in 1964 and had been members of the plan for at least two years. A study group (2,365 men, 2,791 women) and a control group (2,643 men, 2,914 women) were designated by a random process. Members of the study group were urged to have a "multiphasic health checkup" annually. Members of the control group were not urged to have the checkups, but they could have them if they wished. The checkups included,

Table 4-5. Cumulative Mortality from Selected Causes in the Kaiser Health Plan Study of Multiphasic Health Checkups

Cause of death	Sixteen-year cumulative mortality per 1,000	
	Study	Control
Cancer of the colon and rectum	2.3 (12)[a]	5.2 (29)
Cancer of the breast (women)	4.1 (21)	4.3 (24)
Hypertension; hypertensive heart disease; hemorrhagic cerebrovascular disease with hypertension	4.7 (24)	7.2 (40)
Cancer of the bronchus and lung	8.6 (44)	7.6 (42)
Lymphohematopoietic cancer	4.3 (22)	1.8 (10)
Ischemic heart disease	30.2 (155)	27.3 (151)
Suicide	4.9 (25)	2.0 (11)
All causes	113.9 (585)	116.1 (643)

Source: Friedman et al (1986).
[a]The value in parentheses is the number of deaths.

among other tests, electrocardiography, sphygmomanometry, chest x-ray, mammography for women at least 48 years old, and physical examination. Furthermore, Papanicolaou smears were recommended for all women, and sigmoidoscopic examinations were recommended for both men and women who were at least 40 years old. After the study had been in progress for 16 years, 84% of the screened group had had at least one multiphasic checkup, compared to 64% of the control group. Members of the study group had had a mean of 6.8 and a median of six check-ups per subject, and members of the control group had a mean of 2.8 and a median of one check-up per subject.

The Kaiser investigators compared the experience of the study and control groups with respect to outpatient medical service utilization, frequency of hospitalization, disability as reported by mail survey of the subjects, and mortality. Overall, the differences between the study and control groups were small. Only the findings on mortality are discussed here.

Table 4–5 gives the cumulative mortality from several diseases during the 16 years of observation. For all causes combined, mortality was nearly identical for the study and control groups. Cumulative mortality was lower in the study than the control group for cancer of the colon and rectum, and for hypertension and related diseases. On the other hand, mortality was higher in the study group for lymphohematopoietic cancer and suicide. Surprisingly, the cumulative mortality from breast cancer was essentially the same in the two groups.

Cancer of the colon and hypertension are diseases for which screening may be a useful control measure. Therefore, the investigators explored the positive findings for these diseases. One factor to take into account is that subjects may have had diagnosed, before entry, some of the diseases for which screening was done. Dales et al reported "no study-control group difference in mortality from hypertension, hypertensive heart disease, and hemorrhagic stroke preceded by hypertension" in subjects not known to be hypertensive at the start of the study. In contrast, the 11-year cumulative mortality from those causes was 5.8 per 1,000 in the study group, and 17.7 per 1,000 in the control group, among subjects who *were* hypertensive at entry. This finding indicates that it was the continuing observation and treatment of previously diagnosed hypertensives, rather than the early detection and treatment of new cases, that resulted in the mortality difference. This conclusion is supported further by the observation of only a modest study-control difference in the frequencies of new diagnoses of hypertension and in prescriptions of antihypertensive medication (Friedman et al, 1986).

The difference in cumulative mortality from cancer of the colon or rectum is intriguing but the extent to which sigmoidoscopic screening was responsible for it is unclear. The incidence of colorectal cancer was substantially lower in the study group than in the control group. This difference in incidence could not be explained by more frequent removal of colorectal polyps in the study group. In fact, the frequencies of polyps in the two groups were virtually equal. Furthermore, the frequency of sigmoidoscopy was not much greater in the study group than in the control group. By use of the most optimistic assumption on the value of treating sigmoidoscopically-detected colorectal cancer, the study-control difference on sigmoidoscopic exposure would have accounted for only one colorectal cancer death (Selby et al, 1988). Thus, it seems unlikely that the screening program was responsible for the 56% difference in colorectal cancer mortality that was observed. Furthermore, it is plausible that chance variability (Friedman et al, 1986), or perhaps some unrecognized bias, was responsible for part or all of the mortality difference observed. The results for lymphohematopoietic cancer and suicide give some indirect support to this idea. The cumulative mortalities observed for these causes were in the opposite direction but similar in size to the values for colorectal cancer. Since the screening program almost certainly did not cause lymphohematopoietic cancer or suicide, these differences must be regarded as the consequences of unknown factors or chance (Morrison, 1985).

The failure to observe a beneficial effect of screening for cancer of the breast in the Kaiser study might be explained in several ways. First, there were 25 diagnosed cases of breast cancer in the study group at the start of the experiment, compared to 16 cases in the control group. This difference would reduce the apparent value of screening, and the report does not compare the cumulative mortality from breast cancer between study and control groups with these cases removed. Second, the difference in the frequency of examinations between study and control groups was probably smaller in the Kaiser study than in the HIP study. Third, as Dales et al (1979) pointed out, the subjects in the Kaiser study were relatively young; the beneficial effect of screening is uncertain for such women. Fourth, the number of women in the Kaiser study was only about one-tenth the number in the HIP study. Therefore, the precision of the Kaiser data is relatively low, and a beneficial effect of screening may not have been observed as a result of chance variation. Finally, the identification of breast cancer cases and deaths was probably less complete in the Kaiser than in the HIP study.

PLANNING

An experimental study of screening is likely to be a long, complex and expensive undertaking. It is important to create a design that will give useful information for current disease-control efforts and that will also provide a foundation for additional productive research. Compromises will have to be made, since there are certain to be many more questions regarding issues such as screening frequency, combinations of tests, and the ages of screenees than there will be resources to answer them. One of the most important practical questions is this: How many people should be studied, and for how long, in order to provide a reasonably precise estimate of the effect(s) of the screening program(s) to be evaluated?

A study of screening for almost any disease must be large in order to be informative. This is necessary because the only subjects who potentially benefit from screening are those who have disease detected by screening before symptoms would develop; such subjects are likely to be only a small fraction of the total screened. In the HIP study, only about two cases of preclinical breast cancer were discovered per 1,000 examinations. Twenty thousand women had 62,000 examinations in order for only 132 women to be treated early. The cost of large studies places upper limits on their size. On the other hand, a small size increases the chance that a true beneficial effect will be overlooked, and much of the expense and effort wasted. A study that is too small could even be counterproductive; a useful screening procedure might be discarded unnecessarily.

The number of subjects who should be enrolled depends on the

Table 4–6. Expected One-year Cumulative Mortality from Breast Cancer ($\times 10^5$) in Women Eligible for Screening by Year after Entry and Age at Entry

Year after entry	Age at entry (years)							
	35–39	40–44	45–49	50–54	55–59	60–64	65–69	70–74
1	0.8	1.6	3.3	4.6	6.2	8.1	8.7	10.3
2	3.1	6.0	11.5	15.2	18.9	23.1	25.7	28.5
3	6.2	12.2	20.9	27.7	31.7	36.4	41.0	45.0
4	9.9	18.6	30.4	39.8	44.0	48.6	54.5	61.9
5	13.8	24.4	39.0	50.2	55.4	60.0	66.4	76.3
6	17.4	30.5	46.4	58.8	64.8	70.4	76.8	88.9
7	21.0	36.4	52.8	66.6	72.4	79.2	86.3	100.7
8	24.9	41.8	58.0	73.4	78.9	86.3	94.1	111.4
9	29.1	46.7	62.7	79.2	85.2	92.5	101.4	119.6
1–9[a]	126.2	218.2	325.0	415.5	457.5	504.6	554.9	642.6

[a]For a relatively rare disease, the total cumulative mortality is nearly equal to the sum of the time-specific values.

expected cumulative mortality from the disease in the unscreened group or control group during the planned follow-up period, the hypothetical reduction in the probability of death that the new program of screening and early treatment, if effective, would bring about, and the desired precision (usually expressed as the power of a study to reject the null hypothesis of no screening effect) in estimating that difference.

The cumulative mortality expected in unscreened persons following entry into a screening program can be determined from expression (2–1). This method is related to procedures described by Morrison (1985) and Moss et al (1987). The results for breast cancer given in Table 4–6 were derived by use of incidence and case-fatality data from the Surveillance, Epidemiology, and End Results (SEER) program (Young et al, 1981; L Ries, written communication, 1987; Morrison et al, 1988). Since breast cancer is a relatively rare cause of death, the one-year cumulative mortalities are good numerical approximations of mortality rates. Based on this table it can be determined, for example, that ((218.2 + 325.0 + 415.5 + 457.5)/4) = 354 deaths from breast cancer (in the absence of other causes of death) would be expected in a group of 100,000 women, with equal proportions at ages 40 to 44, 45 to 49, 50 to 54 and 55 to 59, who were eligible for screening and who were followed for nine years.

Based on data from the SEER program (Young et al, 1981), the one-year age-specific cumulative mortality from breast cancer in US women is estimated as 12.9 per 100,000 (ages 35 to 39 yr), 22.5 (40 to 44 yr), 42.4 (45 to 49 yr), 62.0 (50 to 54 yr), 79.2 (55 to 59 yr), 92.9 (60 to 64 yr),

105.5 (65 to 69 yr), and 112.3 (70 to 74 yr). In the early years after entry, the mortality expected in women eligible for screening (Table 4–6) is far below the level in the general population. This large discrepancy underscores the importance of accommodating the fact that persons must be free of diagnosed disease in order to be screened.

Expression (2–1) is helpful in estimating expected mortality only if accurate incidence and case-fatality data are available for the disease of interest. If not, a less refined approach will have to be used. In any event, an allowance should be made for the low mortality from the disease among those eligible to be screened.

Ideally, the anticipated reduction in cumulative mortality would be based on the frequency of screen-detected cases and on their natural history—the proportion that would die during the period of follow-up if early treatment had no effect, and the proportion of these that would *not* die in the same period if screening *were* beneficial. However, such information is usually not available; the lack of it is a major reason that the study is being done. Therefore, the anticipated reduction in cumulative mortality is likely to be chosen on practical grounds—that is, the smallest effect that would be feasible and affordable to demonstrate. The HIP study was designed to detect (with only modest power) a reduction of at least 20%. The anticipated benefit should be consistent with reasonable assumptions regarding the proportion of cases detected by screening, and the effect that early treatment has on the natural history of the disease in the cases detected. The proportion of detected cases will depend on subject compliance and on the frequency of screening. Data related to test sensitivity could be helpful. In the HIP study, it was assumed that two-thirds of the women invited would have the first screening examination and that the detected prevalence of breast cancer at this examination would be numerically twice the incidence rate.

The benefit of a given program depends, of course, on the difference between the diagnostic effects of the screening protocols to be compared. This difference is reflected in the lead-time distribution. A comparison of screening v usual care, as in the HIP study, might lead to greater lead times, and therefore more benefit, than a study that compares, for example, screening with mammography and physical examination v screening with physical examination alone, as in the study in Canada (Miller et al, 1981). The lead-time distribution, or factors associated with it (such as the change in the stage distribution), provides an early indication of whether a given study will ultimately be capable of showing a reduction in mortality in relation to screening. A study in which little or no lead time is generated does not constitute a test of the efficacy of early treatment, and no substantial change in the mortality rate would be expected.

The length of the planned observation period should reflect the natural history of the disease under study. The period should be long enough to permit observation of most or all of the changes in mortality rate brought about by early treatment. In other words, the period should at least encompass the times at which most screen-detected cases would die if they were not treated early. For many cancers, therefore, observation periods of at least five to ten years are appropriate. It is believed that most cases that do not recur within five years of diagnosis are cured; to this five-year period must be added the lead time. Quite long periods, perhaps two or three decades, might be necessary when screening detects early precursor lesions such as dysplasia or carcinoma in situ of the cervix, or colonic adenomas. A long period might also be required to learn whether early treatment is curative or simply postpones disease progression and death. A complete description of the effects of screening may require follow-up until all the experimental subjects have died. As suggested in chapter 3, it may not be necessary to actively follow every screened subject for a long period, but only a group of cases. The cases that must be followed are those that come to attention during the period in which the screening program is having an effect on the time of diagnosis—ie, cases diagnosed within a period corresponding to the longest lead time created by the program. In the HIP study, for example, the effect of screening was confined to cases diagnosed within the first five to seven years of the program.

Table 4–7 gives the power that studies with specified numbers of subjects would provide in the circumstances indicated. The table is based loosely on the HIP and Kaiser studies. In each, two groups of approximately equal size were compared. In the HIP study, the outcome assessed was death from a single disease—breast cancer—and the cumulative probability of the outcome, even after five or ten years of follow-up, was quite low. Therefore, a very large number of subjects was required even though a relatively large proportional reduction in deaths, say 20% to 50%, might be expected from a narrowly focused program of this type. On the other hand, the Kaiser study assessed deaths from all causes. The probability of this outcome is relatively high and the Kaiser study had fewer subjects than the HIP study did. However, it seems unlikely that a screening program, even a multiphasic one, would be able to reduce deaths from *all* causes by as much as 10% to 25%.

In planning studies of the effects of etiologic factors, a common goal is to provide about 80% power with a .05-level two-sided test of significance($Z_\alpha = 1.96$). To meet this goal in studies of screening may require inordinately large numbers of subjects because the difference evaluated is likely to be small, compared to studies of etiology. Therefore, it may be necessary to settle for lower power, and to use less stringent tests

Table 4–7. Study Power in Various Circumstances

Cumulative probability of event without screening	True reduction in cumulative probability of event as a result of screening	Number of subjects[a]	Power[b] if Z_α equals		
			1.96[c]	1.645[d]	1.282[e]
.002	20%	50,000	.18	.28	.41
		300,000	.74	.83	.91
.002	50%	50,000	.84	.91	.96
.005	20%	50,000	.39	.51	.65
		150,000	.83	.90	.95
.005	50%	50,000	.99+	.99+	.99+
.02	10%	10,000	.11	.18	.29
		150,000	.81	.88	.94
.02	25%	10,000	.48	.60	.74
		20,000	.77	.86	.92
.05	10%	10,000	.22	.32	.46
		50,000	.75	.84	.91
.05	25%	10,000	.87	.92	.96

[a]Total number of subjects in two groups of equal size.

[b]The power is the probability that a true difference of a given size will result in an observed difference that is statistically significant with a test at a specified level (eg, .05). The values given were derived using a program by Rothman and Boice (1979). Z_α is the normal deviate corresponding to the desired level of statistical significance.

[c]Corresponds to the customary two-tailed .05 significance level.

[d]Corresponds to a two-tailed .1 level or a one-tailed .05 significance level.

[e]Corresponds to a one-tailed .1 significance level.

of statistical significance, than are customary. The possibility that a study was simply too small must be kept clearly in mind when faced with a negative result.

The proportion of all cases detected by screening increases as the screening intensity increases. As the intensity increases, however, the average number of cases discovered *per examination* decreases. If a program is to be done primarily for service or disease control rather than for research, feasibility and cost considerations may favor relatively infrequent screening. However, certain other factors support frequent screening in a program to be done largely for research purposes.

First, frequent screening reduces the number of people who must be recruited into a study, by increasing the number of cases detected in a group of given size. Although frequent screening leads to a relatively high cost per case detected and a relatively large number of false positives, these costs may be less than those of enrolling more people. The number of screen-detected cases in a group of a given size also increases with the duration of a screening program. However, programs done for research purposes should be kept fairly short in order to provide useful results within reasonable times.

Second, frequent screening may reduce the chance that the screening procedure is discarded as ineffective, since frequent screening tends to lead to the detection of cases earlier than does infrequent screening. This would be an important consideration in studying a procedure that is not already known to be effective.

Therefore, an experimental study of a screening procedure, especially a new one, probably should evaluate screening at the greatest frequency that is likely to be feasible as a service activity. If resources permit, a second regimen of less frequent screening also could be included. For example, a study of fecal blood testing compares groups offered screening yearly, every other year, and not at all (Gilbertsen, 1980). The choice of the lower frequency should be guided by what is already known about the natural history of the disease. The goal would be to select a schedule in which examinations are done relatively infrequently but still often enough to provide a useful level of control.

A study that evaluates two frequencies selected in this way would have the following advantages. First, if any feasible screening frequency is effective in reducing mortality, this design should uncover that fact. Second, it should be learned whether less frequent screening, which is more economical and has fewer adverse effects, also offers substantial benefit. Third, such a design actually provides data on *three* screening frequencies—none (the control group), in addition to the two test frequencies. The three sets of observations might suggest the shape of the relation between the intensity of screening and reduction in mortality. Such data would be useful in future research activities and in making disease control programs as efficient as possible.

Cost is the major drawback to including more than one screened group in an experiment. As mentioned previously, a difference in mortality between participants in two screening regimens probably would be smaller than the overall difference between screened and unscreened people. Therefore, extremely large numbers of subjects might be required to obtain a precise estimate of the relative efficacy of two or more active programs.

Estimates of the relative efficacy of screening at various ages could be useful. Age differences in efficacy might arise as a result of age differences in the detectability of the disease or in its natural history. These relationships cannot be investigated on the basis of age at diagnosis because this is an effect of the screening process. Instead, the experiment must be designed with the desired comparisons in mind. To answer the question of whether breast cancer screening is effective for ages 40 to 49, mortality should be compared between women screened only in this interval and women who are not. If, instead, the problem is to estimate the gain achieved by beginning to screen at age 40 rather than age 50, then mortality should be compared between two groups of women whose observation begins at age 40; screening would start in one group at that age, and in the other group at age 50.

Corresponding arrangements would have to be made to compare the value of different screening procedures. A question as to the relative value of mammography and physical examination should be answered by a study in which each group is screened by only one method. If the problem is to estimate the value of mammography over and above that of physical examination, then both tests should be compared to physical examination alone, along the lines described by Miller (1981).

An experimental study is the most convincing means of evaluating the efficacy of screening in improving health status because an experiment ensures, insofar as possible, that confounding, even by factors that are unknown, does not occur. A confounding factor is any characteristic other than screening and early treatment that is unequally distributed among the study groups and that affects either the incidence of the disease or its prognosis. Thus, a confounding factor ultimately leads to a spurious difference in mortality among the study groups. In an experimental study, differences in mortality may appear, by chance, as a result of confounding, but random allocation of subjects tends to distribute potential confounding factors equally. The larger the study, the less likely are substantial differences in outcome as a result of confounding.

The experimental approach, despite its strength, entails serious economic and practical difficulties. Much greater research support is necessary to mount an experimental compared to a corresponding nonexperimental study.[2] If an experimental study of a screening procedure is to be done at all, it probably would have to be done soon after the procedure is introduced. Once a procedure becomes widespread in medical practice, as the Pap smear has, the natural tendency of screen-detected cases to have apparently favorable courses may make it difficult or impossible to convince providers of medical care, or the public, of the appropriateness of an experiment that would include a control group. And, even if an experiment could be organized, the widespread availability of the procedure could lead a high proportion of the control group to be screened, ultimately causing a misleading negative outcome. It might be possible, for example, to organize an experimental study of frequent v infrequent cytologic screening for cervical cancer, but there might be a real question as to whether subjects assigned to infrequent screening would, in fact, have

cancer attended the program to initiate diagnostic studies. Breast
r mortality among women who were actually screened was similar to
mong women who refused screening. Although the screened women
higher incidence rate, they also had the benefit of early treatment.
arison of breast cancer mortality between women who were screened
ither the refusers, the controls, or a combination of refusers and con-
leads to an underestimate of the benefit of screening for the women
participated unless adjustments can be made for the effects of con-
ding factors.

cause of the comparatively large possibility of uncontrolled con-
ding, the results of a nonexperimental study are subject to more
rtainty of interpretation than the results of a corresponding experi-
tal study would be. The error produced by a given set of unidentified
ounding factors decreases in relation to a protective effect of screen-
as its strength increases. Therefore, nonexperimental approaches are
t useful when the effect of screening is strong.

RRELATION STUDIES

relation or ecologic studies describe the relationship between the
eening frequency and the disease-specific mortality rate of several pop-
tions, or of the same population at different times. Correlation studies
ve been relied on heavily in the evaluation of cytologic screening for
icer of the cervix. The results of these studies are summarized and inter-
eted in chapter 11. Some examples are discussed below.

Two types of geographical correlations of cytologic screening and cer-
al cancer mortality may be distinguished. A "before-and-after" analysis
lates the *change* in cervical cancer mortality to the level of screening area
area. In a before-and-after analysis, each area serves as its own control.
amer (1974) showed a positive association between the frequency of the
ip smear and the decline in cervical cancer mortality from 1950 to 1954
states within the United States (Figure 5–1). "After-only" analyses relate
ie *per capita* screening frequency to subsequent mortality, area by area.
ytologic screening and cervical cancer (or uterine cancer) mortality have
een found to be inversely related in provinces in Canada (Miller, 1986)
nd in health districts in the UK (Murphy et al, 1988).

The before-and-after and after-only types of analysis have different
trengths and weaknesses. There is more uncertainty that confounding fac-
ors can be adequately controlled in an after-only analysis. The causal vari-
bles that link willingness to be screened to risk of cervical cancer are not
ompletely understood. The potential confounding factors that have been

additional screening on their own. In such circumstances evaluation would
very likely have to be done by nonexperimental methods. With respect to
the time that a procedure is introduced, the experimental and nonexperimental approaches are complementary. Experiments usually must be
done early, but most nonexperimental approaches—correlation studies,
retrospective follow-up studies, and case-control studies—require the procedure to have been in use for some time.

NOTES

[1]It seems likely that treatment, if effective, functions similarly whether a case comes
to attention as a result of screening or as a result of symptoms. If so, the HIP study
provided important experimental evidence of the value of surgical treatment in
primary breast cancer.

Is an observed decrease in mortality a result of preventing invasion, lymph node
metastases, or more distant spread? The answers to such questions are not obvious.
Although far from conclusive, data from the HIP study suggest that only a small
part of the reduction in mortality was the result of diagnosis of cancer while noninvasive. Most of the benefit seems to have been derived from the earlier diagnosis
of invasive cases (Table 8–5) (Breslow et al, 1977; Shapiro et al, 1982).

[2]But the total cost to society of a nonexperimental study may match or exceed that
of the corresponding experiment. Furthermore, failure to carry out the appropriate experiment could result in a poor screening policy and long-term adverse
consequences.

5 Assessing the Value of Early Treatment: Nonexperimental Studies

were known, the necessary adjustment could be n
regression, or other methods. However, it is conce
ciation reflects confounding by one or more *unide*
problem of nonexperimental research is that ther
method to assess the possibility that an observed
this way. A report of the Coronary Drug Project R
illustrates this problem well. The group studied the
intended to prevent recurrent heart attacks. There v
ence in outcome between the test group and the unt
However, subjects who complied with the assigned re
tially more favorable prognosis than those who did
ference observed was virtually identical for subjec
treatment and those assigned to placebo. Out of a l
ables investigated, none was found that could explain
compliance and prognosis.

In the HIP study there was no placebo—screening
ment—for the control group. Therefore, breast cance
be compared between study and control group mer
compliance, as heart attack rates were compared in t
Project. Even so, the HIP study does contain evidence
participated in screening generally had better health s
those who did not: Overall death rates, exclusive of b
nearly identical for screened and control groups. \
assigned to the screening program, however, the women
had a death rate from causes other than breast cancer th
half as high as the rate in women who refused screening

On the other hand, women actually screened were at r
of breast cancer (Shapiro et al, 1988). This might have c
women exposed to risk factors selected themselves inter
vertently to be screened, or because women who were hav

In a nonexperimental study, the investigator accepts circumstances as they are, instead of arranging them to suit research needs. The exposure (eg, screening history) is not determined by design but by various factors not under the investigator's control, and there is less assurance in a nonexperimental study, compared to an experiment, that observed differences in outcome are the result of screening and not of other characteristics of study subjects. Either the incidence of the disease or its rate of progression might differ between persons who do, and do not, choose to be screened. Suppose, for example, that people of relatively high socioeconomic status (SES) tend to be screened more often than do people who are less well off, and that people of high SES have a lower incidence, and consequently lower mortality from the disease, as a result of less exposure to some causal agent that is not related to screening:

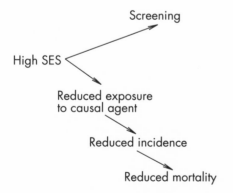

An apparent beneficial relation between screening and mortality might be only the result of social-class factors. If the responsible factor, say, income,

Table 5–1. Rates of Death from All Causes Other than Breast Cancer in the HIP Study

Group	Deaths per 10^4 PY[a]
Total study	56.3
Screened	42.9
Refused	83.7
Control	58.2

Source: Shapiro et al (1988)

[a]Rates during the first five years of the study.

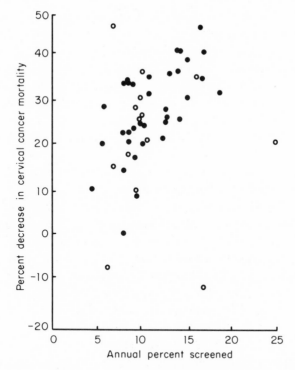

Figure 5-1. Relation of the change in cervical cancer mortality 1950-1954 to 1965-1969 to the annual percent screened, for states in the United States.

Source: Cramer (1974).
Open circles represent states with relatively small populations.

identified may be measured only poorly. However, factors that confound an after-only analysis would not seriously confound a before-and-after analysis unless a change in the distribution of the confounding factor is closely linked to a change in the level of screening.

Mortality from cervical cancer is *inversely* related to social class (Hoover et al, 1975) which, in turn, is *positively* related to screening (National Center for Health Statistics, 1975). Suppose that wealth confounds an after-only analysis: Wealthy women choose to be screened and wealthy women are at low risk of death from cervical cancer for reasons unrelated to screening; the reverse is true for poor women. Wealth would not confound a before-and-after analysis unless a change in the distribution of wealth occurs hand-in-hand with a change in the level of screening.

The after-only method will be relatively accurate after screening in each area has been established at the respective levels long enough for its effect to be roughly constant with time. Then, the geographic correlation between screening and mortality would reflect the value of the screening that was done, provided that confounding factors are controlled. If the intensity of screening is changing, however, the relation of screening and mortality may be difficult to perceive by use of an after-only analysis. On the other hand, the before-and-after method is appropriate when mortality would be expected to be changing as a result of changes in screening intensity. A before-and-after analysis cannot evaluate screening after its effect on mortality has become constant.

The cervical cancer mortality rate has been falling in the United States and a number of other areas, and the rate has declined throughout the period in which use of the Pap smear has become widespread. It is intuitively appealing to attribute the fall in mortality to screening and early treatment. Often, however, simple temporal relations such as this have several plausible explanations in addition to a causal association of screening and the change in mortality. For instance, mortality from cervical cancer was declining long before screening could have had an effect. The increasing frequency of hysterectomy has affected the rates, and there probably are other factors involved as well (Gardner and Lyon, 1977).

Occasionally, circumstances may permit a more informative analysis of the temporal relation of screening frequency and mortality. This is possible when a program of extensive screening is organized in a population where little or no screening was previously done. Then, a close relationship between the establishment of screening activities and the time of a reduction in mortality from the disease is reasonable evidence of the efficacy of the program. Johannesson et al (1978, 1982) described a cervical cancer screening program that appears to have led to a 60% reduction in cervical cancer mortality in Iceland. The program was started in 1964 and was targeted at women aged 25 to 59. By 1977, more than 85% of this group had been screened at least once. The cervical cancer mortality rate of women in this age group was rising until 1970, but then dropped. The cervical cancer mortality rate of older women, screened much less intensively, has shown little change.

In this study, cervical cancer mortality was extremely low following a negative Pap smear, but this observation of a low mortality rate is not evidence in favor of a beneficial effect of early treatment. The trends of incidence and mortality by time after a negative smear depend on the characteristics of the screening test and the natural history of the disease. This information can be used to help establish screening policy, given methods of detection and treatment that are known to be basically effective (chapter 11).

Most correlation studies have an important drawback: Available data on screening frequency consist of averages in groups of people, rather than the actual frequencies with which individuals are screened. Thus, an area in which half the people are screened twice a year would appear to have a similar screening experience to another area in which everyone is screened once annually. As a result of this deficiency, correlation studies may not accurately indicate the relation of screening frequencies for individuals to the reduction in mortality.

On the other hand, correlation studies have a strength not often found in nonexperimental follow-up and case-control studies. Correlation studies involve comparisons of mortality in entire populations that include both screened people and unscreened people who, presumably, could have been screened if they wished. Therefore, a correlation study provides a direct estimate of the impact of screening activities on disease rates in much the same way that an experimental study does, rather than giving a comparison of rates between self-selected screened and unscreened individuals.

Furthermore, a given factor may not have the same confounding effect when the units of observation are groups as opposed to individuals (Blalock, 1964). Social class, a risk factor for cervical cancer, may be a predictor of the probability that an individual woman is screened in a given area, but geographic variation in the level of screening may not reflect socioeconomic factors as much as differences in medical practice from one area to another. In this situation, a geographic correlation study might not be seriously distorted by social class factors.

For most types of screening, the major difficulty of evaluation revolves around measurement of the effectiveness of early treatment. Sometimes, however, this is self-evident or known in advance. For persons to whom therapeutic abortion is acceptable, it is effective in preventing disability from neural tube defects, Down syndrome, etc, among their offspring. In England and Wales, the prevalence of neural tube defects among live births decreased by about 80% from 1964–72 to 1985. Cuckle et al (1989) estimated that half of this decrease was the result of abortions following screening and diagnostic testing, and they concluded that the additional decrease in the birth prevalence of neural tube defects was not the result of screening. (The screening tests that were used most often were ultrasound examination and the maternal serum alpha-fetoprotein (AFP) level. The principal diagnostic tests were ultrasound and amniotic fluid AFP or acetylcholinesterase level.) The remaining prevalence at birth of neural tube defects could be reduced if a higher proportion of pregnant women were screened or if the tests were more sensitive.

FOLLOW-UP AND CASE-CONTROL STUDIES

Conceptually, these types of studies are closely related and provide similar information. They differ with respect to the method of sampling subjects and, sometimes, with respect to data collection and data quality. Breslow and Day (1980, 1987), Kleinbaum et al (1982), Rothman (1986) and Schlesselman (1982) discuss issues in the design and analysis of follow-up and case-control studies.

In a *follow-up study* mortality rates are assessed in groups defined according to screening category. It is also possible to determine the unconditional (observed) cumulative mortality in each group, as in an experimental study. However, the groups compared in a nonexperimental follow-up study usually differ with respect to the distribution of period of follow-up, so that differences in the observed cumulative mortality are likely to be misleading. Therefore, the analysis usually focuses on the rates.

As in an experiment, the outcome of a follow-up study is specified completely by the numbers of deaths and numbers of PY in each exposure group, according to time period, beginning with exposure and continuing indefinitely, or at least until the exposures no longer have effects.

The mortality rates for each follow-up interval may be adjusted for the effects of potential confounding factors that are known, such as social class. Adjustment can be made by stratification and standardization, in which stratum-specific rates are averaged by means of weights that are identical for each of the exposure groups being compared. Standardized rates often do not indicate the experience of any real group. Instead, they are hypothetical rates that would be experienced by groups with the composition specified by the standard set of weights if that group had experienced the observed stratum-specific rates. The standardized rates may be compared by time after the start of follow-up as standardized rate differences (attributable risk) or standardized rate ratios (relative risk). If desired, the time-specific rates may be combined into a single summary figure by further standardization. Other methods of adjustment also are available. The time-specific rates also may be used to derive conditional cumulative mortality by time after the start of observation, or estimated unconditional cumulative mortality given specified death rates from other causes.

Morrison et al (1988) analyzed breast cancer mortality by time among participants in the Breast Cancer Detection Demonstration Project (BCDDP). The BCDDP was a program of five annual screening examinations by mammography and breast palpation that was conducted at 29 centers in the United States. The program began in 1973 and screening ended in 1981. A total of 283,222 women were enrolled. About one-half (51.7%)

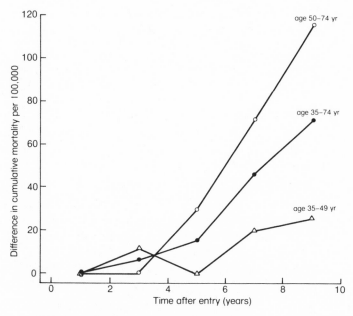

Figure 5–2. Difference between expected and observed mortality from breast cancer by time after entry and age at entry. (Difference = expected minus observed cumulative mortality from breast cancer from entry to the indicated time).

Source: Morrison et al (1988).

of the participants completed all five examinations; 86.7% had two or more examinations. The analysis of breast cancer mortality was based on 55,053 white women who were 35 to 74 years old at entry and who were selected for follow-up.

Mortality in the group that was followed up was compared to expected breast cancer mortality based on data from the Surveillance, Epidemiology and End Results (SEER) program. The expected mortality was derived from incidence rates and CFRs by use of expression (2-1). For the entire nine-year period of follow-up, the observed cumulative mortality from breast cancer was 281.0 per 10,000, which is 80% of the expected value. The observed and expected values are compared by time after entry in Figure 5–2. Mortality from causes other than breast cancer increased rapidly with time in the first few years after entry. The low early mortality reflects the self-selection of relatively healthy women for screening.

The nine-year cumulative incidence of breast cancer in the BCDDP was 1.34 times the expected value. Some women, however, entered the program because of concern about breast disease, family history of breast cancer, or a physician's recommendation. Among women who gave the reason for being screened as "routine" only, the incidence of breast cancer was 1.10 times the expected value, and the mortality from breast cancer was 62.0% of the expected value.

Gilbertsen and Nelms (1978) described a prospective follow-up study of sigmoidoscopic screening for benign neoplasms and cancer of the sigmoid colon and rectum. The incidence and mortality from rectosigmoid cancer in participants in a screening program consisting of annual physical examinations with proctosigmoidoscopy were compared to the incidence and mortality expected in a population of similar age and sex composition. There were 21,150 people who had at least one examination. These subjects were nearly equally divided between men and women at least 45 years old. Subsequently this group had 92,650 additional screening examinations. Any benign lesions that were detected were removed, and cancers that were discovered were treated. Since a total of 113,800 examinations were done, participants had an average of 5.4 examinations. Exact figures on follow-up were not given, but more than 92,000 PY of experience were accumulated, approximately 4.4 years per subject.

During the period of follow-up, which began after the first screening examination, 13 rectosigmoid cancers were discovered by screening and no others were reported. Of these 13 cases, one died postoperatively, another died of what was, apparently, a primary cancer at another site, and the remaining cases were followed for at least five years without known recurrence. The authors estimated that about 90 cases of cancer of the sigmoid and rectum would be expected in 92,000 PY of observation in a group with the age-sex composition of those participating in the screening program, compared to the 13 cases that were observed. Concerning the possibility of volunteer or self-selection bias in the screened group, it was stated that cancers other than those of the sigmoid and rectum occurred at about the expected rates.

Although this report suggests that sigmoidoscopic screening is worthwhile, estimates of the value of annual screening cannot be made with much confidence from the results presented, even if the issue of self-selection is ignored. Gilbertsen and Nelms seem not to have considered cancers diagnosed at the initial screening examination. Some or all of these cases would have come to attention during the observation period if the initial examination had not been done. Twenty-seven cases were found at the initial examination of the 21,150 participants. Thus, as many as 40 cases, rather than 13, might have come to attention if those discovered at the initial screen are included. Furthermore, persons who had colorectal cancer diagnosed between examinations may have been systematically excluded from continued follow-up (Selby and Friedman, 1989).

Similar problems affect the interpretation of the figures given on deaths.

The postoperative death in one of the cases detected at a follow-up screen must be attributed to cancer. Of the first 25 cases detected at the initial examination, 9 died within five years of diagnosis. Assuming that these deaths are all attributable to rectosigmoid cancer, the rectosigmoid cancer mortality rate in the study would be roughly $(9 + 1)/92,000$ PY $= 1$ per 10^4 PY. This rate may be lower than that in the general population, with the same age and sex distribution, but the general population mortality rate is not a suitable comparison figure. Since people known to have cancer must have been excluded from initial screening, the correct comparison value is likely to be substantially less than the death rate from sigmoid and rectal cancer in the general population. There is no obvious way, however, to make an adjustment for the apparent lack of follow-up of cases diagnosed between examinations.

In a *case-control study* (Greenland and Thomas, 1982; Miettinen, 1976; Morrison, 1982a) subjects are identified on the basis of outcome rather than exposure. Thus, the investigator's point of access to an exposure-disease relation is at the end of the sequence rather than at the start. Despite some controversy regarding this supposedly backward design, however, there is nothing illogical about case-control studies. Other things such as data quality and control of confounding variables being equal, a case-control study provides estimates of an exposure-disease association that are just as valid as the corresponding estimates from a follow-up study.

In most modern case-control studies of chronic diseases, the cases are identified on the basis of a disease event, usually a new diagnosis, or death from the disease. Controls are selected concurrently from the living population in which the cases arise. If cases are defined as newly diagnosed patients, controls are selected from well people. In a study of the value of screening in reducing the death rate, cases are defined as deaths from the disease screened for regardless of the means of initial diagnosis, as in an experiment or a nonexperimental follow-up study. This group would include deaths from disease diagnosed as a result of screening, as well as deaths from disease that was first diagnosed following the occurrence of symptoms. Eligible controls would include all living members of the source population—people who never had had the disease, as well as people who had had the disease, whether or not screen-detected.

It may seem strange that people with the disease could be included in the control series. However, in a study concerned with whether or not screening reduces the likelihood of *death*, a living person with the disease is a member of the source population, but is not a case. Furthermore, as a result of early diagnosis by screening and, perhaps, postponement of death by early treatment, a living person with the disease is more likely to have been screened than is someone without the disease. Systematic exclusion of diseased people from the control series would tend to remove screened subjects preferentially, and reduce the apparent size of a true beneficial effect of the screening program.[1]

If the cases and controls are selected concurrently, the controls corresponding to a given case reflect the distribution of PY by screening history in the source population for the period during which the case arose. Define a short period Δt in which the case was identified, and let Δt be short enough so that the number of people in the source population, as well as the distribution of exposure, is constant. Let the number screened be n_s and the number unscreened be $n_{\bar{s}}$. In Δt, the number of PY among screened people is $n_s \Delta t$, and the number among unscreened people is $n_{\bar{s}} \Delta t$. The expected ratio of screened to unscreened controls selected from this population during Δt is $n_s/n_{\bar{s}}$, which is also the ratio of PY in the two exposure groups.

Suppose that the number of deaths from the disease during Δt in screened and unscreened people are, respectively, d_s and $d_{\bar{s}}$. The death rates are $d_s/n_s \Delta t$ and $d_{\bar{s}}/n_{\bar{s}} \Delta t$. In a case-control study, deaths (the cases) would be selected without regard to screening history with a probability of selection P_1. Controls would be selected, also without regard to screening history, with probability P_2. The expected number of exposed and nonexposed cases (Ca) selected would be, respectively, $P_1 d_s = Ca_s$ and $P_1 d_{\bar{s}} = Ca_{\bar{s}}$. Similarly, the expected numbers of controls (Co) would be $P_2 n_s = Co_s$ and $P_2 n_{\bar{s}} = Co_{\bar{s}}$. Therefore, the rates in screened and unscreened people can be expressed, respectively, as

$$\frac{(1/P_1)Ca_s}{(1/P_2)Co_s \, \Delta t} \quad \text{and} \quad \frac{(1/P_1)Ca_{\bar{s}}}{(1/P_2)Co_{\bar{s}} \, \Delta t}$$

The ratio of these rates reduces to

$$\frac{Ca_s/Co_s}{Ca_{\bar{s}}/Co_{\bar{s}}} = \frac{Ca_s Co_{\bar{s}}}{Co_s Ca_{\bar{s}}}$$

which is the familiar *relative odds* (or exposure-odds ratio or cross-product ratio). Thus, the relative odds is an estimate of the ratio of mortality rates, and other things being equal, the relative odds differs from the rate ratio only as the result of sampling variability. It is worth emphasizing that the correspondence of the odds ratio and the rate ratio arises because the sampling fractions of cases and controls do not depend on their exposure, and because the distribution of exposure is constant in the period during which the controls linked to a given case are selected.

The ratio of mortality rates in exposed compared to nonexposed people can be evaluated by the case-control approach even if the sampling fractions of cases and controls, P_1 and P_2, are not known, and in fact, these quantities are not known in the vast majority of case-control studies. If the sampling fractions are known, however, estimates can be made of the rates themselves and their difference, as well as their ratio. (The difference also could be obtained if the rates were known for one of the exposure categories, say the nonexposed.) Typically, the sampling fractions are available in population-based studies, in which all cases arising in a known population are identified ($P_1 = 1$), and controls are selected at random from the same source population, providing for the determination of P_2.

The validity of a case-control study depends on the availability of exposure histories of good and comparable quality for both case and control series. Screening histories might be obtained from records of a health maintenance organization. On the other hand, it may not be possible to obtain screening histories from records, and it might be necessary to interview living cases and controls. In this situation, potential cases could be defined as persons who develop a manifestation (other than death) of disease that is sufficiently advanced to ensure diagnosis even without screening, and thus be past the lead-time interval. For example, cases could be defined as persons who develop symptomatic metastases of cancer. Such persons would include those in whom screening detected an early cancer that later recurred and spread as well as persons with advanced cancer whose disease was first diagnosed following the occurrence of symptoms. Members of the source population without the defining characteristics of a case—advanced illness—would be eligible for the control series. These persons would include those who had had early disease, whether or not screen-detected, that was treated and had not recurred, as well as people who never had had the disease, whether or not they had been screened. The relative proportions screened in the case and control series yield an estimate of the ratio of the rate of development of advanced cancer in screened compared to unscreened people. It is also possible to use a hybrid design in which screening histories are obtained from newly diagnosed cases and from controls (Berwick et al, 1989; Prentice, 1986). The subjects are then followed up. The cases for analysis are those that die subsequently.

Verbeek et al (1984) used the case-control method to evaluate screening for breast cancer in Nijmegen, the Netherlands. Biennial screening with single-view mammography began in 1975. Initially, all women aged 35 to 65 were invited to participate. About 85% accepted the invitation. Subsequently, older women also were offered screening. The report was based on four rounds of screening (through 1981). Of women invited, 65% attended the second screen, 57% attended the third screen, and 53% attended the fourth screen. Forty-six women were identified as cases; these were women who were first diagnosed with breast cancer after their invi-

Table 5–2. Distribution of Screening History in
Case-Control Sets in Study of Effect of Screening
for Breast Cancer

| | Number of controls screened | | | | | | |
Case[a]	0	1	2	3	4	5	Total
Screened	0	0	4	5	8	9	26
Not screened	2	2	4	2	4	6	20

Source: Verbeek et al (1984).
[a]A case was defined as a death from breast cancer.

tation to be screened and who died of breast cancer in the period 1975 to
81. For each case, five controls were selected at random from residents
who were alive at the time that the case died. Controls were matched to
cases by year of birth. Within each case-control set, exposure was considered to be a history of screening in the program before the date of diagnosis of the case. Fifty-seven percent of the cases and 70% of the controls
had been screened. Table 5–2 shows the distribution of screening exposure in the case-control sets. Based on this distribution, women who
accepted the invitation to screening were estimated to have had 0.48 (0.32
to 1.00) times the mortality rate of breast cancer that nonparticipants had.
The investigators were concerned that women who participated in the
screening program might have had a different risk of breast cancer than
nonparticipants. Therefore, they compared the incidence rate of breast
cancer among nonparticipants to the rate in a nearby city where breast
cancer incidence and mortality had been similar to that in Nijmegen and
where no organized screening had been done. With adjustment for age,
the two rates were nearly identical. Thus, participants in screening did not
appear to have been selected in relation to breast cancer risk.

Case-control studies have been done to evaluate screening for other
types of cancer. Oshima et al (1986) used the case-control method to evaluate screening for stomach cancer in Nose town, Osaka Prefecture, Japan.
Persons who were screened were estimated to have had about half the
mortality rate of stomach cancer that nonparticipants had. Ebeling and
Nischan (1987) reported a case-control study of radiologic screening for
lung cancer. There was almost no association between screening and lung
cancer mortality. This finding is consistent with the results of experimental
studies of screening for lung cancer (chapter 4).

Case-control studies of screening for cancer of the cervix are summarized in chapter 11, where methodologic issues in these studies are discussed. These issues include case definition, the difficulty of distinguishing

screening tests from diagnostic tests, the length of the time period during which screening exposure is determined, and the relation of the effect of screening to time since testing.

A central problem in the design and analysis of follow-up and case-control studies of screening is the classification of subjects as to the screening that they have experienced. The next section is devoted to this issue.

CLASSIFICATION OF EXPOSURE TO SCREENING: Because they are based on observations of individuals, follow-up and case-control studies frequently are regarded simply as experiments in which exposure is determined by self-selection instead of random allocation. This would be true if the screening to which subjects are considered to be exposed is determined through a process that is analogous to assignment in an experiment. For example, there might be several medical care organizations in an area, each offering a different program of screening for a given disease. Then, mortality from the disease could be compared among subscribers to the various organizations, beginning at their dates of enrollment.

It is more likely, however, that it will be necessary to classify screening exposure on the basis of actual experience—the number and timing of screening examinations taken. This is a fundamental difference between experimental studies, in which the exposure category is known from the moment of assignment, and those nonexperimental studies in which the exposure is known only after it has occurred. This difference complicates the design and analysis of follow-up and case-control studies of screening and mortality or advanced morbidity.

The difficulty is that the initial diagnosis of the disease can affect the extent of exposure. A diagnosis, whether or not the result of screening, precludes the possibility of subsequent screening. A diagnosis is, in addition, a strong predictor of mortality from disease. If the relation between diagnosis and subsequent screening experience is not properly accommodated, erroneous estimates of the disease-control value of screening may be obtained. People who are screened are expected to be at lower risk of death from the disease compared to the source population, even if early treatment is not effective. As shown on pages 35 to 40, this difference may be quite large.

An analysis might relate risk of death to the number of screens taken (at a given intensity). However, persons must remain free of diagnosed disease during the period of testing in order to experience many examinations. Consequently, a history of multiple screens may appear to be associated with a lower risk of death than will a single screen. Furthermore, the more intensively screening is done (during a given interval), the more likely it is that an existing case of preclinical disease will be detected, since a case that is a false negative on one screen is increasingly likely to be detected as the intensity of subsequent screening increases. People who have experienced intensive screening for a given period without having the disease discovered are less likely than people screened negatively but less intensively to have undiagnosed preclinical disease or to die of the disease later, even if early treatment has no value. Therefore, a history of intensive screening may appear to be associated with a lower risk of death than a history of less intensive screening.

For some time, it has been known that employed groups experience lower mortality than do the populations from which they are drawn. This difference is the "healthy-worker effect" (Monson, 1980). Ill people might not be able to seek employment or to meet the requirements of a new job, and people who become ill might have to leave their jobs (Enterline, 1976; Fox and Collier, 1976). The counterparts of these circumstances may give rise to a "healthy-screenee effect." People known to have the disease are not eligible to enter a screening program or to continue to be screened.

In the HIP study, about 39% of the women invited to screening completed all four examinations. There were 69 cases of breast cancer diagnosed in this group during the fifth through seventh years after entry (cumulative incidence $= 0.00578$). This is the period that began *after* the fourth examination and ended at about the time that the total numbers of diagnosed cases became equal in the study and control groups. The cumulative incidence during the fifth through seventh years in the control group was 0.00736. Women who elected to have a given examination in the HIP study had a higher risk of breast cancer than did the corresponding women who refused screening (Walter and Day, 1983; Shapiro et al, 1988). Nonetheless, the measured incidence in the fifth through seventh years was lower in the women who had four previous negative examinations than it was in the controls because the screening led to the early identification of preclinical cases of breast cancer that otherwise would have been diagnosed during that period.

During the fifth through seventh years after entry, the cumulative mortality from breast cancer was 0.00034 in the women who had completed four negative screens, compared to 0.00128 in the entire group of controls. This difference cannot have been the result of the early treatment of breast cancer, which could have occurred only following positive tests. The deaths in the screened group must have been derived entirely from cases diagnosed only after the fourth (and last) examination, while the deaths in the control group are derived from cases diagnosed at any time after entry. If the women who had four negative examinations were given another examination at the start of the fifth year, and mortality in this group were compared to mortality during the same period in the entirely unscreened

Table 5–3. Mortality Rate from All Causes (Screened and Control Groups Combined) According to Number of Examinations Taken in the Kaiser Study of Multiphasic Screening

Number of examinations	Crude mortality rate (deaths per 1,000 PY)	Age-standardized mortality ratio
0	8.6	1.00[a]
1	6.4	.76
2	4.7	.52
3	5.4	.59
4+	4.6	.41

Source: Dales et al (1979).
[a]Reference group.

controls, a large difference would be observed even if the fifth screen were entirely ineffective.

Table 5–3 gives some additional data from the Kaiser study of multiphasic health checkups (Dales et al, 1979). The death rate from all causes is related to the number of checkups that subjects, either study or control, actually took. The rate decreased markedly with the number of examinations. Subjects who took four or more had only about half the death rate of those who took none. Healthy-screenee bias is likely to have influenced these results. Among those who took a given number of examinations, mortality was *higher* in the study group than in the control group. This difference implies that there also was an effect of self-selection for screening (Friedman et al, 1986).

The problem of healthy-screenee bias does not arise if the screening exposure of subjects is classified according to their assignment in an experiment. In the HIP study, members of the study group who had breast cancer diagnosed at the first screening examination could not have established a pattern of annual screening. Nonetheless, these cases were classified as having been assigned to four examinations at intervals of a year, and their experience was consistent with their assignment up to their times of diagnosis. Similarly, the key to avoiding healthy-screenee bias in a nonexperimental study is to classify cases according to patterns with which the screening that they experienced was consistent up to their times of diagnosis.

In an experiment, the protocol defines a screening schedule so that its effects can be evaluated. The schedule must specify the time of at least one examination. The schedule may also give the times of additional examinations. Screening tests include those that result in a diagnosis. Time may refer to age or to the calendar. When time refers to the calendar, it usually includes a specification of age, as well. For example, an initial screening examination might have been offered in 1975 to persons who were at least 50 years old.

In a nonexperimental study, the screening experience of each subject may be described by a series of dates on which tests were done. In order to analyze this experience, the investigator should refer it to a screening schedule. Of course, the schedule must be one that is encompassed by the experience of the study population. A number of choices of schedule to be evaluated may be possible because of the variability of individual screening exposures in uncontrolled circumstances.

A screening schedule may be described by a series of ages or times, eg, 1, 2, 3, ... These points, referred to as *listed times,* need not be equally spaced, but they are considered to be spaced at yearly intervals to simplify the discussion. The following list gives some types of schedules.

a. Initial examination at the *first* listed time without consideration of further screening (eg, screening at age 50 with or without further screening).

b. Initial examination at *any* listed time without consideration of further screening (eg, screening at age 50 or greater with or without further screening). This schedule is equivalent to allowing the first listed time in schedule (a) to vary from person to person.

c. Initial examination at the first listed time followed by additional screening at listed times (eg, screening at age 50 with annual screening to be continued indefinitely).

d. Initial examination at any listed time followed by additional screening at subsequent listed times (eg, screening at age 50 or greater with annual screening to be continued indefinitely).

e. Single examination at a specified listed time but no further screening (eg, a single examination at age 50).

f. Single examination at any listed time but no further screening (eg, a single examination at age 50 or greater).

A person who is eligible to begin being screened has had no previous diagnosis of the disease, has reached the time (age) at which screening is available according to the specified schedule, and has not been screened before. In some circumstances, a person screened negatively much earlier might be considered to be eligible. This issue is discussed below.

A simple means of avoiding healthy-screenee bias was described by Morrison (1985, pages 112–113). Exposure is defined at a single point, as in schedule (a) or (b). Eligible subjects are restricted to those neither screened nor known to be diseased before the first listed time, the start of observation. The subjects are then classified according to whether or not they were screened at the start, without consideration of further screening. The determination of deaths and PY begins at the first listed time, and subsequent mortality rates are compared between the groups. The overall effect of screening is a function of these rates according to time from the start of observation. This method may also be used to evaluate the second or later examination in a series among those persons eligible (those who have negative results on all specified earlier examinations and no diagnosis up to the scheduled time of the examination to be evaluated).

In analyses based on schedules (a) or (b), persons first screened at some time after the start of observation are classified as unscreened at the start. If such persons were considered to be screened, healthy-screenee bias would be created. Unlike persons never screened, those screened relatively late would have had to be free of diagnosed disease up to the time of screening. As a result, their subsequent mortality would be relatively low even if early treatment were not beneficial.

This approach is illustrated by use of data from the HIP study. The analysis corresponds to schedule (a). Screened women were considered to be those who actually took at least the initial examination that was offered. For these women, the first listed time was considered to be the date of the first examination. The assigned control group was used for comparison. For this group, the first listed time was considered to be the date of entry. Table 5–4 gives the number of breast cancer deaths and the number of PY by year of observation, for screened and control women. In this example, breast cancer deaths were based on the certified cause of death because this procedure would be used in typical case-control and follow-up studies. The results differ slightly from those based on the special review of cause of death that was done in the HIP study.

Various summary measures may be used to compare the experiences of the groups. The standardized mortality ratio (SMR) is one such measure that is well suited to the discussion that follows. The SMR is the observed number of deaths in the exposed group divided by the number expected based on the experience of the comparison group, assuming that the comparison group has the same proportional distribution of PY according to stratification variables as the exposed group (Rothman, 1986, pp. 45–49). In this example, the only stratification variable is time. The observed SMR over all seven years is 0.677 (Table 5–4). (Traditionally, the ratio of observed to expected deaths is multiplied by 100 in the SMR. This constant factor is ignored here.) The SMR in the example is virtually identical to the crude ratio of mortality rates (0.678) because the PY are distributed similarly by time in the two groups. Breast cancer incidence in the HIP study was somewhat higher in women actually screened than it was in controls. Therefore, this nonexperimental analysis is likely to underestimate

Table 5–4. Computation of Standardized Mortality Ratio (SMR) and Mantel-Haenszel (MH) Estimates Comparing Breast Cancer Mortality between Women Who Had At Least One Screening Examination and Control Women in the HIP Study

Year of observation		Screened	Control	Components of SMR[a,b] a	Components of SMR[a,b] $\frac{bc}{d}$	Components of MH estimate[a,c] $\sum \frac{ad}{n}$	Components of MH estimate[a,c] $\sum \frac{bc}{n}$
1	Breast cancer deaths	2	2	2	1.323	.602	.398
	PY	20,163.5	30,485.0				
2	Breast cancer deaths	4	5	4	3.314	1.203	.997
	PY	20,100.5	30,324.5				
3	Breast cancer deaths	5	10	5	6.637	1.503	1.995
	PY	20,013.0	30,153.0				
4	Breast cancer deaths	3	18	3	11.962	.901	3.593
	PY	19,909.0	29,959.5				
5	Breast cancer deaths	9	23	9	15.302	2.702	4.594
	PY	19,795.0	29,754.0				
6	Breast cancer deaths	14	26	14	17.312	4.202	5.196
	PY	19,665.5	29,534.0				
7	Breast cancer deaths	13	27	13	17.989	3.901	5.398
	PY	19,520.5	29,298.0				
1–7	Breast cancer deaths	50	111	50	73.839	15.014	22.171
	PY	139,167.0	209,508.0				

[a]For a follow-up study, let
  a = no. of screened cases (deaths);
  b = no. of unscreened cases (deaths);
  c = PY among screened persons;
  d = PY among unscreened persons.
For a case-control study, let
  a = no. of screened cases (deaths);
  b = no. of unscreened cases (deaths);
  c = no. of screened controls;
  d = no. of unscreened controls.

[b]In a case-control study, cases and controls are selected without respect to exposure. Controls reflect the exposure (screening) distribution of PY that is the source of the cases. Therefore, each term a and (bc/d) in a case-control study is the same (except for random variation) as it would be in the corresponding follow-up study.

[c]The analysis of a matched case-control study may be thought of as being based on a separate stratum for each matched set. The components of the MH estimate of the rate ratio given in

the protective effect of screening, compared to what the effect would be in an experiment with full compliance.

Another useful summary measure is the Mantel-Haenszel (MH) estimate of the rate ratio. In a follow-up study with large strata, the MH estimate is equivalent to a standardized rate ratio in which each weight of standardization is the stratum-specific product of the PY in the exposed and comparison groups divided by their sum. These weights differ from those of the SMR by the multiplicative factor, (PY among exposed persons)/(total PY).

A case-control analysis of this HIP experience would involve identification of the deaths (cases) according to the period after the start of observation in which the deaths occurred, and selection of a sample of living subjects (controls) in each period. The cases and controls are classified as to whether or not they had been screened initially. If the numbers of cases and controls in each stratum are sufficiently large, the SMR can be calculated as $\Sigma a/\Sigma(bc/d)$, where the sums are made over the strata. As indicated previously in this chapter, the distribution of exposure among controls reflects that of the PY in the respective period. Therefore, the SMR in a case-control study is the same, aside from chance variation, as it would be in the corresponding follow-up approach, because the sampling fractions of cases and controls cancel.

---

the table are those that would be expected in a study with 1:1 matching of cases and controls ($n = 2$). There are four possible sample outcomes for each stratum.

1. $a = 1, b = 0, c = 1, d = 0$ $ad/n = 0, bc/n = 0$
2. $a = 1, b = 0, c = 0, d = 1$ $ad/n = \frac{1}{2}, bc/n = 0$
3. $a = 0, b = 1, c = 1, d = 0$ $ad/n = 0, bc/n = \frac{1}{2}$
4. $a = 0, b = 1, c = 0, d = 1$ $ad/n = 0, bc/n = 0$

An exposed case ($a = 1$) accounts for a positive contribution to $\Sigma ad/n$ if the matched control is not screened (outcome 2). The expected number of such contributions is equal to the number of screened cases times the expected proportion of controls that are unscreened. This porportion is equal to the PY among unscreened persons divided by the total PY in the source population from which the cases and controls are selected. Thus, the $\Sigma ad/n$ for year 5 was calculated as $9 \times (\frac{1}{2}) \times (29754.0/49549.0) = 2.702$. Similarly, the expected number of positive contributions to $\Sigma bc/n$ is equal to the number of unscreened cases times the expected proportion of controls that are screened. The $\Sigma bc/n$ for year 5 was calculated as $23 \times (\frac{1}{2}) \times (19795.0/49549.0) = 4.594$.

For years 1–7:

$$\text{Crude rate ratio} = \frac{50/139,167.0 \text{ PY}}{111/209,508.0 \text{ PY}} = .678$$

$$\text{Standardized Mortality Ratio (SMR)} = \frac{50}{73.839} = .677$$

$$\text{Mantel-Haenszel (MH) rate ratio} = \frac{15.014}{22.171} = .677$$

The MH method is useful for the analysis of case-control studies in which the numbers of subjects in the strata are small, including matched designs. A matched study may be thought of as one in which a separate stratum is created for each set of a case and its matched controls. The MH estimate is calculated as $\Sigma(ad/n)/\Sigma(bc/n)$, with the sums made over the sets. The term n is the number of subjects (case plus controls) in each set. Table 5–4 shows the results that would be expected in the HIP example, if one control were selected for each case. In this example, the MH estimate of the mortality ratio is virtually equal to the SMR because the factor d/n (the case-control equivalent of PY among exposed persons/total PY) is nearly constant from stratum to stratum.

Since the age at initial screening varied, the HIP data might also be viewed as an example of schedule (b): The age at the time of the initial examination, or lack of it, could correspond to a schedule of initial screening at any listed age from 40 to 64. If the probability of accepting the invitation to be screened were related to age, then age would be a confounding factor, since it is also related to breast cancer mortality. This possibility could be evaluated by further stratifying the data in Table 5–4 according to age at the start of observation.

The type of case-control analysis shown in Table 5–4 is often described as a *case-control within a cohort* or a *nested* case-control study, derived in this instance from an experiment. As in an experiment or a nonexperimental follow-up study, the periods of observation were defined with respect to the time that exposure status was initially determined.

In contrast, observation periods in typical case-control studies are defined with respect to age. Thus, cases (deaths) and controls are identified in a series of age strata. The data from each of these strata may be used to obtain estimates of the effect of screening that is begun at earlier listed ages that may vary (schedule (b)). If there is substantial variation in age at the start of screening in the source population, then cases and controls at a given age include the experience of separately identifiable cohorts first screened (or not screened) 1, 2, 3, . . . years previously.

Among cases and controls 50 years old, for example, exclude anyone screened or diagnosed before age 45. Those screened at age 45 are considered exposed. Those not screened at age 45 (but possibly screened later) are considered not exposed. The data shed light on the effect of screening in the sixth year of observation. Similarly, those 50-year-old cases and controls who were initially screened at age 46, or who were not diseased and not screened at age 46 or earlier, provide information on the effect of screening in the fifth year of observation. (Note that persons first screened at age 46 would have been considered as unscreened at age 45). Data from the same age stratum of subjects may also provide information on shorter or longer periods of follow-up after the start of screening. If the effect of screening as measured by the mortality ratio does not depend on the age at which screening is begun, then the effect of screening, overall or by period of observation, is appropriately summarized over all age strata. Otherwise, summary estimates over the period of observation may be derived separately according to age at first examination.

Cases and controls at a given age might be assembled in matched sets. A given set furnishes information on the value of an initial screening examination at the earliest age at which any member of the set is screened, provided that this occurs at an age that is no later than the earliest age at which any member of the set has the disease diagnosed. The age at which the first member of the set is screened is considered to be the first listed time for that set. The second or subsequent members of the set to be screened, if any, are considered to have been unscreened at the listed time even if the later examinations are done earlier than any diagnoses in the set. Sets in which all members were screened at the same age, or in which no member is screened, do not contribute to estimation of the relation between screening and mortality.

It may seem strange that members of a set who were screened at different ages should be considered as *discordant* with respect to exposure. Compared to persons screened at the first listed time, however, those screened later may have a low expected mortality at a given age at observation. Such persons must not have had the disease diagnosed up to the time at which screening was done, while persons screened at the earlier specified time but not later could have developed the disease during the ensuing interval. To consider persons screened at different ages as *concordant* for screening exposure fails to take account of this difference in risk, which may introduce healthy-screenee bias. The size of the bias would depend on the difference in ages at screening.

In the analyses presented so far, subjects who were screened at the start of observation may or may not have continued to be screened. Furthermore, subjects classified as unscreened at the start may have been screened later. As no allowance was made for changes in exposure status, the apparent effect of screening may not correspond to the effect of a specified schedule, assuming full compliance. It is possible to estimate the effect of repeated screening, assuming full compliance, while avoiding healthy-screenee bias. Flanders and Longini (1990) proposed the use of a model that links incidence and case-fatality functions. The general problem of estimating the effect of sustained or repeated exposures on mortality has been addressed by Robins (1986, 1987). The discussion that follows shows how stratification and adjustment may be used to provide control of healthy-screenee bias in follow-up and case-control studies.

In brief, the approach is to use only deaths among cases that occur in persons who continue to be screened according to the schedule of interest [eg, schedule (c)]. The observations are then adjusted to give an estimate of the effect of screening under the assumption that all persons who began to be screened according to the specified schedule complete the scheduled screening, unless the disease was diagnosed. The approach is roughly analogous to the traditional life table, which estimates mortality or survival under the assumption that all persons who come under observation complete the entire period of follow-up.

A person is considered to be exposed according to a given screening schedule from the time that the first examination is taken, as specified in the schedule, until the person's screening stops conforming to the schedule, in the absence of a diagnosis. If a group's conformance with a given screening schedule is perfect, the total number of deaths from the disease is the sum of deaths among cases diagnosed at each scheduled examination and in the respective intervals that follow. If conformance is imperfect, the numbers of deaths from the disease among cases with specific screening experiences (eg, exactly one test completed, exactly two tests, etc) may be adjusted for conformance at the respective exams to give the total number of deaths that would be expected assuming full conformance. Thus, every screened individual contributes to the analysis up to the point at which he stops following the schedule. Suppose that the specified schedule is annual screening beginning at age 50. Someone who is screened at age 50 and age 51, and who fails to be screened at age 52 (although eligible) is withdrawn from the exposed group at age 52. A person who has a diagnosis while following the specified schedule is classified as exposed. Diagnoses in persons who have stopped following the schedule are ignored.

For this type of analysis, conformance must be evaluated for each scheduled screening examination. Since all screened persons take the first examination, conformance at the first examination is 100%. Conformance at a given examination after the first is defined as the proportion (of all persons who took the first examination) who took the later examination, divided by the proportion eligible to take it (those who were alive, took all intervening scheduled examinations, took no unscheduled examinations, and had no previous diagnosis of the disease). Suppose that there is 50% conformance at the second examination. For a given number eligible, full conformance would imply that there would be twice as many cases detected by screening, and twice as many cases diagnosed among screened persons after the second examination as were observed. Therefore, the corresponding numbers of deaths among these cases also would be increased by a factor of two.

Consider estimating the effect of four screens for breast cancer at annual intervals (the HIP protocol). Women who took the first examination contribute data on deaths among cases diagnosed from the first examination up to the time that they became eligible for the second examination. The second examination could be taken only by women who did not have breast cancer diagnosed up to that point, and who were still alive. Therefore, women who took the second examination contribute data on deaths among cases diagnosed from the second examination up to the time that they became eligible for the third examination, and so on.

Women who failed to take a scheduled examination were defined as not complying with the schedule as of the time of the missed examination. Thus, women who were considered to be noncompliers as of the second examination included those who took only the first examination as well as those who took the first and third or fourth, but not the second, examination. All examinations taken by women who were complying with the schedule were considered to have been taken as planned, at 12-month intervals.

The proportions of initially-screened women who, if eligible, were screened at each successive annual examination, are designated as p_2, p_3, and p_4. The proportion whose histories conformed to the initial scheduled examination, at the start of observation, is defined as $p_1 = 1$. In general, these proportions may be abbreviated as p_j, where the subscript j is an index of the order of the respective screening examination. These proportions may be thought of as being derived from a life table in which persons are entered at the time of an initial screening examination. Persons are subsequently withdrawn at the time that they fail to take a scheduled examination. In a follow-up study, the p_j's may be derived from the actual numbers of subjects who took specific examinations. In a case-control study, the p_j's may be estimated from the control series.

Table 5–5 gives additional details from the HIP study: the numbers of women under observation in each period who took specified numbers of examinations, the proportions (p_j's) of initially-screened women who complied with subsequent examinations, and the numbers of breast cancer deaths according to the number of screening examinations taken and whether the respective cases were diagnosed during the period of compliance with the screening schedule. The p_j's were derived from the screening experience of the living population during each year of follow-up.

In the fifth year of observation, for example, there were two breast cancer deaths among women who took only one examination in sequence, limiting the deaths to those among cases diagnosed within a year of the first examination (ie, up to the time at which the woman became eligible for the second examination); there were two breast cancer deaths among women who took two examinations in sequence, limiting the deaths to

Table 5-5. Distribution of Number of Screening Examinations Taken, Proportions of Initially Screened Women Complying with the HIP Protocol, and Numbers of Breast Cancer Deaths According to Compliance

Year of observation	Number of screens[a]	Number of Women[b]	Proportion complying (p_j)[c]	Total	Breast cancer deaths[d] Diagnosis while complying	Breast cancer deaths[d] Diagnosis while not complying
1	1	20,163.5	1.000	2	2	na
2	1	4,163.0	1.000	4	3	1
	2	15,937.5	.793	0	0	na
3	1	4,130.0	1.000	1	0	1
	2	2,202.5	.794	2	1	1
	3	13,680.5	.684	2	2	na
4	1	4,100.5	1.000	1	0	1
	2	2,170.0	.794	1	0	1
	3	1,677.0	.685	1	1	0
	4	11,961.5	.601	0	0	na
5	1	4,066.5	1.000	3	2	1
	2	2,150.0	.795	2	2	0
	3	1,651.5	.686	3	2	1
	4	11,927.0	.603	1	1	na
6	1	4,023.5	1.000	6	6	0
	2	2,131.0	.795	2	1	1
	3	1,634.5	.687	2	0	2
	4	11,876.5	.604	4	4	na
7	1	3,981.5	1.000	4	2	2
	2	2,107.0	.796	4	1	3
	3	1,620.0	.688	1	0	1
	4	11,811.5	.605	4	4	na

[a]Women who took at least the first examination are further classified according to the number of screens taken according to the HIP protocol. This categorization corresponds to the extent of participation in a version of schedule (c). The maximum number of screens that could have been taken at a given time of observation is the highest number in the respective section of the table. For example, women who were complying fully with the schedule would have had three screens as of year 3.

[b]Average number during the interval. As the intervals are one year long, these numbers are equivalent numerically to PY.

[c]The proportion complying (p_j) describes the screening distribution of the source population, with respect to the schedule, during a specified year of observation. Consider year 5 as an example. Initially screened women may be classified according to their continued compliance with the schedule of four screens at annual intervals [schedule (c)]. These proportions were determined from the corresponding numbers of women under observation. Thus, of all women who had at least one examination and who were under observation during year 5, the proportion who took all four screens was estimated as $p_4 = 11927.0/(11927.0 + 1651.5 + 2150.0 + 4066.5) = 0.603$. As the incidence of breast cancer is low, the numbers who could not have been reexamined because of a previous diagnosis have only small effects on the p_j's. For simplicity of presentation, no allowance was made for these numbers.

[d]These are the breast cancer deaths during the indicated year of observation among women in the respective exposure categories. Initially screened women may be classified according to their continued conformance with a schedule of four screens at annual intervals [schedule (c)]. Deaths in cases diagnosed among women who were complying are defined as those in which the diagnosis occurred within a year of taking screens 1 through 3, or at any time (through year 7) after taking examination 4. Deaths in cases diagnosed among women who were not complying are defined as those in which the diagnosis occurred a year or more after taking screens 1 through 3 in women who did not take the next scheduled examination.

those among cases diagnosed within a year of the second examination (ie, up to the time at which the woman became eligible for the third examination). Similarly, in the fifth year there were two breast cancer deaths among women who took three examinations according to the protocol, and there was one breast cancer death among women who took all four examinations.

There were 20,188 women who took the first screening examination. If all these women continued to be screened according to the protocol, the breast cancer mortality rate among screened women in the fifth year of observation would be estimated as follows:

Deaths attributable to cases diagnosed within 1 year after first examination = 2

Deaths attributable to cases diagnosed within 1 year after second examination = $2 \times (1/p_2 = 1.258) = 2.516$

Deaths attributable to cases diagnosed within 1 year after third examination = $2 \times (1/p_3 = 1.458) = 2.916$

Deaths attributable to cases diagnosed from fourth examination through 7 years after entry = $1 \times (1/p_4 = 1.658) = 1.658$

Thus, 9.090 total deaths, and a breast cancer mortality rate of 9.090/ 19,795.0 PY = 46 per 100,000 PY would be expected in year 5 among screened women if there had been continued full compliance by the women who took at least one examination. Table 5–6 illustrates the method of estimating the effect of screening on breast cancer mortality, assuming that screened women complied fully with the scheduled screening. For all seven years of follow-up, the SMR, compared to unscreened women, is 0.589 (Table 5–6). The corresponding MH estimate also is 0.589.

It is possible to estimate the effect of less than four screens. For example, the value of a program of a single screening examination [schedule (e) or (f)] would be of interest. For this analysis, women who took exactly one examination would be defined as conforming to the schedule. Women who took more than one examination would be defined as nonconformers beginning at the time of any subsequent examination. There were relatively few women who took exactly one examination, and there were only ten deaths among cases diagnosed in this group from one year after the first examination through seven years after entry. Therefore, the estimated effect of a single examination derived from the HIP data would be very imprecise.

Series of p_j's also could be chosen arbitrarily in order to estimate the potential effects of screening programs with hypothetical degrees of conformance. The p_j's could be either greater or less than the observed values.

Table 5–6. Computation of Standardized Mortality Ratio (SMR) and Mantel-Haenszel (MH) Estimates Comparing Breast Cancer Mortality between Women Who Complied with HIP Protocol and Control Women

Year of observation		Screened[a]	Control	Components of SMR[a]		Components of MH estimate[b]	
				a	$\dfrac{bc}{d}$	$\sum \dfrac{ad}{n}$	$\sum \dfrac{bc}{n}$
1	Breast cancer deaths	2 × 1.000	2	2.000	1.323	.602	.398
	PY	20,163.5[c]	30,485.0				
2	Breast cancer deaths	3 × 1.000 +0 × 1.261	5	3.000	3.314	.902	.997
	PY	20,100.5	30,324.5				
3	Breast cancer deaths	0 × 1.000 +1 × 1.259 +2 × 1.462	10	4.183	6.637	1.257	1.995
	PY	20,013.0	30,153.0				
4	Breast cancer deaths	0 × 1.000 +0 × 1.259 +1 × 1.460 +0 × 1.664	18	1.460	11.962	.439	3.593
	PY	19,909.0	29,959.5				
5	Breast cancer deaths	2 × 1.000 +2 × 1.258 +2 × 1.458 +1 × 1.658	23	9.090	15.302	2.729	4.594
	PY	19,795.0	29,754.0				

6	Breast cancer deaths	6 × 1.000	26	13.882	17.312	4.167	5.196
		+1 × 1.258					
		+0 × 1.456					
		+4 × 1.656					
	PY	19,665.5	29,534.0				
7	Breast cancer deaths	2 × 1.000	27	9.868	17.989	2.961	5.398
		+1 × 1.256					
		+0 × 1.453					
		+4 × 1.653					
	PY	19,520.5	29,298.0				
1–7	Breast cancer deaths	43.483	111	43.483	73.839	13.057	22.171
	PY	139,167.0	209,508.0				

[a] In calculating the "a" terms that contribute to the numerator of the SMR, the numbers of screened cases contributing to each "a" term are multiplied by the respective $1/p_j$ as explained in the text (pages 122 to 123).

[b] Adjustment by the respective $1/p_j$ is made to each contribution to the ad/n terms that are added to give the numerator of the MH estimate. The effect of this adjustment is to yield the terms that would be expected if every person who began to be screened according to the defined schedule continued to be screened, if eligible, up to the age at observation. For year 5, the contributions to ad/n were calculated as follows.

$$2 \times (\tfrac{1}{2}) \times 29754.0/49549.0) \times 1.000 + 2 \times (\tfrac{1}{2}) \times (29754.0/49549.0) \times 1.258$$
$$+ 2 \times (\tfrac{1}{2}) \times (29754.0/49549.0) \times 1.458 + 1 \times (\tfrac{1}{2}) \times (29754.0/49549.0) \times 1.658 = 2.729$$

[c] In principle, the PY among screened persons should be adjusted upward as a result of decreased deaths owing to full compliance with screening. In practice, this correction is likely to be trivial.

For years 1–7:

Crude rate ratio = $\dfrac{43.483/139,167.0 \text{ PY}}{111/209,508.0 \text{ PY}} = .590$

Standardized Mortality Ratio (MR) = $\dfrac{43.483}{73.839} = .589$

Mantel-Haenszel (MH) rate ratio = $\dfrac{13.057}{22.171} = .589$

The type of analysis described may be done by use of the case-control approach. As in the follow-up analysis, the components of the numerator of the SMR—the observed numbers of cases—would be multiplied by the factors $1/p_2$, $1/p_3$, and $1/p_4$. In the MH method, the components of the numerator—the ad/n—are multiplied by the respective $1/p_j$ to give the result that would be expected if there had been full conformance with the screening protocol.

An analogous method may be used to accommodate changes in status from unscreened to screened. A person is considered not exposed from the time at which eligibility begins until the time at which the first examination is done. A person who has a diagnosis while not exposed is considered permanently not exposed. Define a series of q_j's that describe the probability that a person who is unscreened at a specified listed age continues to remain unscreened at subsequent listed ages. Deaths among cases diagnosed among unscreened persons would be adjusted by the q_j's to estimate what the numbers of deaths would be if there had been no subsequent screening among persons who were classified as unscreened at a specified listed age.

In nonexperimental studies, subjects may be stratified in order to control confounding factors that are associated independently with both screening and mortality or advanced morbidity. If a series of p_j's is to be used to adjust results for incomplete conformance, the p_j's should be determined within strata of confounding factors for which the p_j's are known, or reasonably assumed, to be constant. If age is a confounding variable, the p_j's should be determined within age strata if the p_j's vary with age. If the p_j's are constant with age, it would be reasonable to use all available data to obtain relatively stable estimates of them. An age-stratified analysis that makes use of common p_j's implies that the probability of beginning to be screened varies with age (as does mortality from the disease) but that, once screening is begun, the probabilities of continuing to be screened do not depend on age. These comments apply to both matched and unmatched case-control designs, as well as to follow-up studies. With most matched designs, and some unmatched designs, it will be impossible to obtain useful estimates of the p_j's within individual strata, ie, the matched sets. Therefore it will be necessary to assume that the p_j's are constant over at least some of the strata. For example, subjects might be matched by both age and income. It might be assumed that the p_j's depend on income but not age. If so, the p_j's would be estimated over age strata, but within income strata, of the controls.

As pointed out in chapter 2, the cumulative effect of screening on mortality is easiest to perceive if the analysis is limited to cases that come to attention during the period of the diagnostic effect of screening, ie, while the incidence is elevated by screening. T_m may be defined as the duration of this period (see chapter 3). In the HIP, for example, T_m occurred about five to seven years after the start of screening, or about two to four years after the close of screening. In a nonexperimental study, T_m may be determined as it would be in an experiment, by comparison of the cumulative incidence in the screened and unscreened groups. A study concerned exclusively with mortality, however, would not provide a direct estimate of T_m because nonfatal cases would not be ascertained. If a goal of a study is to make use of T_m in estimating the effect of screening on mortality, two choices are available. The first is to obtain a series of estimates of the effect of screening using different possible values of T_m, (eg., basing mortality on cases diagnosed within five, seven, or ten years of the start of screening). The largest proportional effect of screening is presumed to be obtained at the value of T_m that would have been observed. The second is to obtain data on T_m directly by ascertaining incident cases as well as deaths. This can be done in either case-control or follow-up studies. This method has the advantage of providing data on the lead-time distribution, as well as on the effect of screening on mortality.

Case-control studies are likely to be done in settings in which screening is ongoing, rather than being limited in duration as it would be in an experimental program. Ongoing screening usually is repeated at intervals shorter than the maximum length of the preclinical phase. Therefore, participants in ongoing screening continue to experience its diagnostic effects; all deaths among such subjects would occur in cases diagnosed within T_m. A person who was screened, but who failed to take a later examination as scheduled, may be withdrawn from the screened group at the time that participation stops. Such a person, however, should not be reconsidered as unscreened until reaching the age that corresponds to T_m after the last examination taken. Compared to truly unscreened persons, the incidence of the disease is reduced before this age in nonconformers with repeated screening. If they are considered prematurely to have returned to unscreened status, the observed mortality in persons classified as unscreened will be too low. Unless information on T_m is available, subjects who stop following a schedule of repeated screening should not be considered to return to unscreened status.

There may be some circumstances in which the procedures outlined can be relaxed, and in which a simpler approach would not lead to serious error. This would be the case if the screening patterns of interest are established a long time before the outcome is to be assessed, so that subjects can be placed in an expsoure category that by itself does not predict risk. For example, the development of advanced breast cancer in a group of women aged 50 or older might be related to the frequency of breast self-examination of those women when they were in their twenties. The purpose would not be to evaluate breast self-examination in young women but to use this exposure as an indicator of continuing the practice at older ages. Early breast cancer or other precursor conditions that affected the frequency of self-examination in the twenties probably would be unrelated to the occurrence of advanced breast cancer two or more decades later.

Other types of simplification also may be possible, but little is known about the effects of various choices on the size of healthy-screenee bias. Note that correlation studies would not be affected much by healthy-screenee bias; the diseases for which screening is done are sufficiently rare that their occurrence will have little impact on the screening frequency in a population.

NOTES

[1]Weiss (1983) pointed out that "there seems to be a certain intuitive appeal to a different approach to selecting controls, one that would select *only* persons with disease that is not advanced." Presumably, this approach is attractive because early-stage and late-stage cases may have similar distributions of incidence risk factors that are also determinants of screening and so may confound comparisons of cases and mostly nondiseased controls. As Weiss indicates, however, early-disease controls are more likely than late-disease cases are to have been screen-detected even if early treatment offers no benefit. Thus, in contrast to a control series from which diseased people have been excluded, the use of early disease controls is likely to suggest a benefit even if none exists.

6 The Clinical Course of Screen-detected Disease

There are several important questions that need to be answered concerning the prognosis of patients whose disease is brought to attention by screening. What sort of clinical course are these patients likely to experience? To what extent are differences in the prognosis of screen-detected v routinely diagnosed cases the result of the diagnostic effects of screening, and to what extent is early treatment responsible?

The clinical course of screen-detected disease often appears quite benign. In the HIP study, for example, about 13% of the screen-detected cases died within five years of diagnosis compared to 40% of cases in the control group (Shapiro et al, 1988). This large difference should not be taken to represent the effect of early treatment alone; the observed case fatality of screen-detected disease also is affected by lead time, and possibly by prognostic selection (a tendency to have a clinical phase that is unusually long or short). Shapiro et al (1982) assumed the lead time of all screen-detected cases to be one year. With this correction, the five-year cumulative case fatality of screen-detected cases was 19%. If this correction was adequate, and if there was no important prognostic selection, then early treatment actually reduced case fatality to 19/40 = 48% of the value in the control group, rather than 13/40 = 33%.

Refer again to Figure 2–6 and to the corresponding hypothetical case-fatality rates in Table 6–1. If there is no screening (example (a)), the five cases experience a total of $2 + 2 + 1 + 0.5 + 1 = 6.5$ PY of observation in the clinical phase. Since all five patients die, the observed case-fatality rate (CFR) is 6/6.5PY = 0.77 per PY. If screening is done, three cases are detected. If there is no prolongation of life as a result of early treatment, ie, no reduction in the overall mortality rate [example (b) of the table], the observed CFR of these three cases is $3/(5 + 4 + 2)$PY = 0.27 per PY, only 35% of the CFR of 0.77 for all five cases if no screening is done, and

Table 6–1. The Effects of Early Treatment, Lead Time, and Prognostic Selection on the Fatality of Screen-detected Cases, Based on Figure 2–6

Group	Case-fatality rate (CFR)
a. All cases	5/6.5PY = 0.77/PY
b. Screen-detected cases *if not detected early*	3/5PY = 0.6/PY
c. Screen-detected cases, no benefit from early treatment	3/11PY = 0.27/PY
d. Screen-detected cases, reduced mortality from early treatment	2/11PY = 0.18/PY
e. Cases not detected by screening	2/1.5PY = 1.33/PY

Effect of early treatment on CFR = c − d = 0.09/PY
Effect of lead time on CFR = b − c = 0.33/PY
Effect of prognostic selection on CFR = a − b = 0.17/PY (or e − b = 0.73/PY)

only 20% of the CFR of cases not detected by screening $[2/(1 + 0.5)PY = 1.33$ per PY]. Obviously, the apparently favorable clinical course of the screen-detected cases is not a beneficial effect of early treatment. The entire difference is a consequence of early detection and a tendency of screening to find cases that would have long clinical phases even if no screening were done. If early treatment *does* lead to some prolongation of life [example (c)], the CFR of screen-detected cases is reduced still further, to $2/(5 + 4 + 2)PY = 0.18$ per PY, for the first five years of observation. A comparison of this figure with either the overall CFR of 0.77 in the unscreened group or the rate of 1.33 among routinely diagnosed cases in the screened group greatly overstates the actual benefit of a 20% reduction in the overall mortality rate stemming from a 33% reduction in cumulative fatality among cases treated early (pages 37 to 39).

A beneficial effect of early treatment leads to a decrease in the number of deaths from the disease, the numerator of the CFR. The CFR in screen-detected cases is 2/11PY if early treatment is beneficial, and 3/11PY if it is not. (In addition, if the period of observation were extended past five years, the PY in the denominator of the CFR would be increased because the cured case remains under observation.) The lead time due to early detection increases the PY of observation, decreasing the observed CFR, of screen-detected cases. Thus, the CFR of screen-detected cases [example (b)] is 3/11PY; the CFR of the *same* cases but not detected by screening [example (a)] is 3/5PY. Prognostic selection is indicated by the fact that even if there is no screening, the three cases that would be screen-detected have longer clinical phases than do the remaining two.

These differences suggest a means of separating the effects that early treatment, lead time, and prognostic selection have on the CFR. This analysis is possible because the length of follow-up of a group of cases detected by screening at the start of an experiment corresponds to the duration of the experiment. Therefore, the timing of the accumulation of lead time and the decrease in mortality in a screened population can be related to the experience of screen-detected cases. In a given period after screening, a reduction in the number of deaths (the numerator of the CFR) can only be the effect of early treatment (or chance). Therefore, this reduction (ie, two deaths v three, in Figure 2–6) can be estimated by comparing the numbers of deaths in the screened group [example (c)] and an otherwise comparable unscreened group [example (a)]. The effect of lead time is to increase the number of PY in the denominator of the CFR. The number of people experiencing lead time in a given period, and the total amount of lead time, are given by the lead-time distribution. In the example, there is a total of 6 PY of lead time. The benefit of early treatment and the lead time as reflected in these numbers can be removed from the CFR of screen-detected cases. Thus, the observed CFR is 2/11PY; the CFR with the effects of treatment and lead time removed is $(2 + 1)/(11 - 6)PY = 3/5PY$, which is the same as the CFR of the three cases in example (a) that *would* have been detected by screening had screening been done. Prognostic selection can be evaluated by comparing the CFR, 0.6 per PY, with the overall CFR of cases in the unscreened group, 0.77 per PY, and with the CFR of cases in the screened group that were not detected by screening, 1.33 per PY. The lower CFR of screen-detected cases is the effect of prognostic selection. These results are summarized in Table 6–1.

Although the effects of early treatment, lead time, and prognostic selection can be separated as outlined, it is important to emphasize that this method does not obviate the need to compare mortality rates between entire screened and unscreened populations in order to evaluate early treatment. In fact, the analysis presented in this chapter depends on information derived from this type of comparison. To assess early treatment by use of case-fatality data alone, it would be necessary to know the distribution of lead times gained by the screen-detected cases being studied and the effect of prognostic selection on case fatality by time after diagnosis. This information can be derived from experimental screening programs and from some types of nonexperimental comparisons of mortality between screened and unscreened persons. The methods described cannot be applied to a series of screen-detected cases whose experience cannot be related to the corresponding source population of screened persons (which includes cases not detected by screening, and nondiseased persons) and an otherwise comparable population of unscreened persons.

Aron and Prorok (1986) made use of a measure of case fatality in which PY of cases begin to accumulate at the time of assignment to screened or control groups, irrespective of the time of diagnosis. This measure of case fatality is not affected by lead time or prognostic selection. On the other hand, this measure provides no more information on lead time or prognostic selection than do comparisons of mortality rates between screened and control groups. The Aron and Prorok measure of case fatality differs only by the absence of PY of non-cases in the denominator from a disease-specific mortality rate. In a large randomized study with equal-sized screened and control groups, the PY of non-cases will be virtually equal in the two groups. Therefore, comparisons of mortality or the Aron-Prorok case fatality will reflect the same trends. The numerical values of the comparisons will differ only because of the presence of a virtually constant factor in the denominators of the mortality rates but not the case fatalities.

The methods suggested by the example are now developed more generally in the context of a one-time screening program and are then extended to programs of repeated screening (Morrison, 1982b). Again, refer to the situation described in chapter 3. A group free of clinical disease is offered a single screening examination and then followed up. An unscreened, but otherwise identical, group is followed up as well. The notation below corresponds to that introduced in chapter 3. However, the analysis is based on prevalent numbers alive instead of cumulative numbers diagnosed because the CFR in a given interval after entry applies to cases alive and under observation at the start of the interval.

Let

C_{os} = number of cases detected by the screening examination

$C_{i.}$ = total number of diagnosed cases in the screened group alive at time i after entry, whether or not these cases were detected by screening

$\overline{C}_i$ = total number of diagnosed cases in the unscreened group alive at time i after entry

In addition, define the following quantities for the screened group:

C_{is} = number of screen-detected cases alive at time i after entry

D_{is} = total number of deaths from the disease among C_{is} during the interval from i to $i + \Delta t$

$D_{i.}$ = total number of deaths from the disease among $C_{i.}$ during the interval from i to $i + \Delta t$ whether or not the deaths occur among screen-detected cases

N_i = number of persons, diseased or not, alive at time i after entry

Finally, in the unscreened group, let

$\overline{D}_i$ = number of deaths from the disease among $\overline{C}_i$ during the interval from i to $i + \Delta t$

CASE-FATALITY RATE: The CFR is the ratio of the number of deaths from the disease observed in a series of cases to the amount of person-time the series experiences during the period of observation. The CFR has the same numerator as the mortality rate in a given period but a different, smaller, denominator. The denominator of the mortality rate is the total person-time experienced by both ill and well people. The denominator of the CFR is the person-time experienced only by ill people. The CFR is an estimate of the force of mortality to which cases, rather than all members of the screened population, are exposed. For a short period Δt during which the number of people at risk of death is essentially constant, the amount of person-time in the denominator of either the CFR or the mortality rate can be factored into the number of people under observation, and the length of the interval. Therefore, the

$$\text{CFR} = \frac{\text{Number of deaths}}{\text{Number of cases}} \times \frac{1}{\Delta t}$$

For all cases in the screened group, the CFR in the interval from i to $i + \Delta t$ is

$$\frac{D_{i.}}{C_{i.}} \times \frac{1}{\Delta t}$$

The mortality rate in the entire screened group during the same period is

$$\frac{D_{i.}}{N_i} \times \frac{1}{\Delta t}$$

For cases detected by screening, let the CFR be

$$R_i = \frac{D_{is}}{C_{is}} \times \frac{1}{\Delta t}$$

In a one-time screening program, the time after diagnosis for all screen-detected cases is the same as the time after entry for everyone in both the screened and unscreened groups, whether or not diseased. That is, at time T after screening, all screen-detected cases have been followed for T years, and everyone else in both groups also has been followed for T years. Therefore, the components of the mortality rate of screen-detected cases, D_{Ts} and C_{Ts}, can be related to any reduction in deaths in the screened population before and during the respective interval Δt, and to any increase in the prevalent number of cases diagnosed in the screened, compared to the unscreened, group.

The prognosis of cases often has been measured by the proportion that survives for at least a given period after diagnosis, typically five years. The effects of causes of death other than the one of interest may be removed. The probability that a screen-detected case will survive the disease for at least a given period of time after diagnosis is estimated readily from the R_i's. If the R_i is constant with time, the cumulative proportion of cases that dies from diagnosis to time T after diagnosis given survival of other causes of death, is

$$q_T = 1 - \exp(-R_i T)$$

If the case-fatality rate varies with time, the cumulative proportion that dies from diagnosis to T is

$$q_T = 1 - \exp\left(-\sum_{i=0}^{T-1} R_i \Delta t\right)$$

(Rothman, 1986). If the fatality rates among cases in the first five years after diagnosis were, respectively, 0.15, 0.1, 0.1, 0.095, and 0.09, then q_T would be

$$1 - \exp[-(0.15 + 0.1 + 0.1 + 0.095 + 0.09) \times 1] = 0.41$$

The q_T is the conditional cumulative case fatality from the disease. The proportion that survives the disease from diagnosis to time T is $p_T = 1 - q_T$. This value is equivalent to the T-year survival of a series of cases at risk of death only from the disease of interest, not from other causes.

EFFECT OF EARLY TREATMENT

If screening and early treatment lead to reduced mortality from the disease among the people screened, there are fewer deaths from the disease during some Δt's in the group offered screening than in the comparison group. For an interval in which this benefit is realized, the screened group experiences $(\overline{D}_i - D_i)$ fewer deaths than the unscreened group.

Cases that benefited during previous time periods may still be alive during a given Δt. The number of such cases depends primarily on the cumulative difference in deaths from the disease between the screened and unscreened populations, or

$$\sum_{i=0}^{T-1} (\overline{D}_i - D_i)$$

However, this number may be reduced by deaths from other causes. If the disease that is the object of the screening program causes only a small fraction of the total mortality, as would be true for cancer of a particular site, the proportion of benefited cases that survive other causes of death is approximated well by the proportion of the screened population that survives *all* causes of death. Therefore, the number of cases that live to T as a result of reduced mortality during previous time periods can be taken to be

$$\sum_{i=0}^{T-1} (\overline{D}_i - D_i) \frac{N_{T-1}}{N_i}$$

which is abbreviated as $\Sigma \, \Delta D_T$. (If the groups under observation were subject to death only from the disease for which screening is done, the number of cases in the screened population alive as a result of earlier treatment would simply be the cumulative excess of diagnosed cases minus those experiencing lead time.)

The effect of early treatment can be removed from the case-fatality rate observed during a given Δt by increasing the numerator of the rate by $\overline{D}_T - D_T$, the number of additional deaths that would have occurred during the interval if there had been no therapeutic value in screening, and decreasing its denominator by $\Sigma \, \Delta D_T$, the number of additional cases that would not have been alive and at risk during the interval except as a result of early treatment.

If the subscript b indicates that the effect of early treatment has been removed, then

$$R_{Tb} = \frac{D_{Ts} + (\overline{D}_T - D_T)}{C_{Ts} - \Sigma \, \Delta D_T} \times \frac{1}{\Delta t} \tag{6-1}$$

The quantity R_{Tb} is what the CFR of screen-detected cases would have been if early treatment did not prolong life. Compared to the mortality rate of routinely diagnosed cases, R_{Tb} will still be reduced as a result of lead time, and R_{Tb} also may reflect prognostic selection. By using the exponential relation given previously, the T-year survival free of the benefit of early treatment is estimated as

$$p_{Tb} = \exp \left(- \sum_{i=0}^{T-1} R_{ib} \, \Delta t \right)$$

For the Δt corresponding to T, the reduction in case fatality attributable only to early treatment is

$$B_T = R_{Tb} - R_T \tag{6-2}$$

EFFECT OF LEAD TIME

Cases detected by screening are not at risk of death from the disease (except as an adverse effect of treatment) until the remainder of the pre-clinical phase has passed. However, cases experiencing lead time are included in the denominator of the observed fatality rate of screen-detected cases (R_i) and the CFR with the effect of early treatment removed (R_{ib}), and thus reduce them compared to what they would be if there were no lead time. The contribution of lead time to the reduction in case fatality will be especially large immediately after screening. Then all, or nearly all, of the screen-detected cases would be experiencing lead time. With continuing observation, the proportion of cases experiencing lead time diminishes, and the CFR increases correspondingly.

The lead time can be removed from R_i by subtracting from the denominator the number of cases experiencing lead time. When this value is derived from the prevalent numbers of cases, it must be corrected for the number of cases in the screened group alive because of earlier treatment. Thus,

$$l_i = C_{i.} - \overline{C}_i - \Sigma \, \Delta D_i$$

Applying this correction to R_{Tb} leads to

$$R_{Tbl} = \frac{D_{Ts} + (\overline{D}_T - D_{T.})}{C_{Ts} - \Sigma \, \Delta D_T - (C_{T.} - \overline{C}_T - \Sigma \, \Delta D_T)} \times \frac{1}{\Delta t}$$

$$= \frac{D_{Ts} + (\overline{D}_T - D_{T.})}{C_{Ts} - (C_{T.} - \overline{C}_T)} \times \frac{1}{\Delta t} \tag{6–3}$$

The R_{Tbl} is what the fatality rate of screen-detected cases would have been during a given interval if the cases under observation had not been diagnosed early and had not received any benefit from early treatment. An estimate of T-year survival can be computed from R_{Tbl} as for R_{Tb} and R_T.

For the specified interval, the reduction in case-fatality attributable to lead time (LT) is

$$LT_T = R_{Tbl} - R_{Tb} \tag{6–4}$$

EFFECT OF PROGNOSTIC SELECTION

Even after adjustment for lead time and the effect of early treatment, the clinical course of screen-detected cases and routinely diagnosed cases may differ. The screening test itself may tend to detect cases that will have a favorable or unfavorable prognosis. This process is described in this chapter under the heading *length-biased sampling*. (Note that the healthy-screenee bias described in chapter 5 concerned the comparatively low mortality rate that would be expected in persons eligible to be screened, or rescreened, because persons with a previous diagnosis are not eligible for screenings. The present discussion concerns the prognosis of diagnosed screen-detected cases.)

If there is no prognostic selection acting at time T after diagnosis, the fatality rate of screen-detected cases with early treatment and lead-time effects removed, R_{Tbl}, is equal to the mortality rate of cases T years after diagnosis in an unscreened population, $E\{R_T\}$. The quantity

$$W_T = E\{R_T\} - R_{Tbl} \qquad (6-5)$$

measures the extent of prognostic selection.

If prognostic selection is the result of length-biased sampling, the cases that are not screen-detected have the opposite change in prognosis from those that are; a comparison of R_{Tbl} to the fatality rate of interval cases would lead to a larger difference than is given by expression (6–5). On the other hand, persons who choose to be screened may, if they become ill, have prognoses that are relatively good, or perhaps poor. In this situation, interval cases might have a case fatality similar to that of screen-detected cases with the effects of treatment and lead time removed.

The quantity W_i may be positive or negative. If screening attracts health-conscious people who would tend to have favorable clinical courses, regardless of lead time or benefit of early treatment, expression (6–5) would tend to be positive. If all members of the population offered the screening program are actually screened, this form of self-selection bias would not occur. Then, the W_i's reflect only the detection of relatively rapidly or slowly progressing lesions by the screening test.

REPEATED SCREENING: The major complication introduced by repeated screening is that the start of observation of both screened and unscreened groups—the time of the first examination—does not coincide with the time of diagnosis for all screen-detected cases, since cases will be detected at examinations other than the first one. Therefore, the CFR at time T after the start of the program cannot be interpreted simply as the CFR at T years after diagnosis. Instead, the analysis probably must consider the screening program as a unit.

At T years after the start of a screening program with repeated examinations, R_T, the overall fatality rate of screen-detected cases (in the respective Δt), can be viewed as a weighted average of fatality rates of cases detected at each examination. Each of these rates would correspond to a time after diagnosis equal to T minus the interval from the start of the program to the screen at which detection occurred. The weight would be the number of cases from the respective examination that are prevalent at T. Thus,

$$R_T = \frac{\sum_j C_{T-j,s} R_{T-j}}{\sum_j C_{T-j,s}} \tag{6-6}$$

where the j's are the times from the start of the program to the screen at which detection occurred; j equals zero for cases diagnosed at the first examination. The effects of early treatment and lead time can be removed from R_T as in a one-time program. A measure of the effect of prognostic selection on the clinical course can be obtained by subtracting the resulting R_{Tbl} from

$$E\{R_T\} = \frac{\sum_j C_{T-j,s} E\{R_{T-j}\}}{\sum_j C_{T-j,s}} \tag{6-7}$$

There are circumstances in which it would be possible to evaluate the effects of early treatment, lead time, and selection bias on CFRs for specific intervals after diagnosis. Imagine a program of $1, 2, \ldots, k, \ldots$ examinations at times $t_1, t_2, \ldots, t_k, \ldots$. For cases diagnosed at the kth screening examination, the time after diagnosis is $i - t_k$. If observations are available on populations screened exactly k times and exactly $k - 1$ times, the analysis can proceed as it would for a one-time screening program. Take the population screened $k - 1$ times as "unscreened," and the population screened k times as "screened." If $t_k = 0$, so that i becomes the time after the kth screen, expressions (6-1) to (6-5) apply to cases diagnosed at the kth screen.

The methods presented here are illustrated with data from the HIP program (Table 6-2). Cases diagnosed through seven years after entry are included. As in chapter 3, the numbers of cases are expressed as averages over one-year periods.

The prevalent number of cases detected by screening, C_{is}, increases for the first few years as a result of the repeated examinations. For the third through seventh years, the number of breast cancer deaths in the screened group, $D_{i,}$, is smaller than the corresponding number in the control group, $\overline{D}_i$, reflecting the value of early detection and treatment.

Table 6-3a presents the crude case-fatality rates (R_i), the rates with the effects of early treatment and lead time removed (R_{ib}, R_{ibl}), and the reductions in the rate attributable to early treatment and lead time. Table 6-3b illustrates the computations. Because the HIP study involved repeated

Table 6–2. Basic Data for Analysis of the Fatality Rate of Screen-Detected Cases[a]

Completed years after entry (i)	Study group					Control group	
	Number of screen-detected cases[a] C_{is}	Number of screen-detected cases alive because of early treatment[b,c] $(\Sigma \Delta D_i)$	Total number of cases C_i	Number of breast cancer deaths among C_{is} D_{is}	Number of breast cancer deaths among C_i D_i	Number of cases[b] $\bar{C}_i$	Number of breast cancer deaths $\bar{D}_i$
1	37.5	−1.0	45.4	2	6	30.3	2
2	72.1	−3.4	104.8	2	5	86.9	6
3	91.5	−2.9	150.9	2	6	128.0	11
4	110.8	7.5	198.3	0	7	165.3	19
5	123.0	18.5	243.3	4	15	205.6	25
6	118.9	29.6	284.9	4	19	246.6	32
7	112.6	36.0	320.3	3	23	288.3	29

[a]Based on the HIP study.

[b]Average number during the interval.

[c]For simplicity, $\Sigma \Delta D_i$ has not been adjusted for deaths from other causes.

Table 6–3a. Analysis of the Fatality Rate of Screen-detected Cases

Completed years after entry (i)	Observed case-fatality rate[a] R_i	Case-fatality rate with effect of early treatment removal[a] R_{ib}	Reduction in case fatality from early treatment[a] $B_i = R_{ib} - R_i$	Number of cases experiencing lead time[b] l_i	Case fatality rate with effects of early treatment and lead time removed[a] R_{ibl}	Reduction in case fatality from lead time[a] $LT_i = R_{ibl} - R_{ib}$	Case fatality rate in control group[a]
1	.053	−.052	−.105	16.1	−.089	−.037	.066
2	.028	.040	+.012	21.3	.055	.015	.069
3	.022	.074	.052	25.8	.102	.028	.086
4	.000	.116	.116	25.5	.154	.038	.115
5	.033	.134	.101	19.2	.164	.030	.122
6	.034	.190	.156	8.7	.211	.021	.130
7	.027	.117	.090	−4.0	.112	−.005	.101

[a]Deaths per PY.
[b]Average number during the interval.

Table 6–3b. Computation of Quantities for First Year ($i = 1$) in Table 6–3a

$$R_1 = \frac{D_{1s}}{C_{1s}} \times \frac{1}{\Delta t} = \frac{2}{37.5} \times \frac{1}{1 \text{ yr}} = 0.053 \text{ per PY}$$

$$R_{1b} = \frac{D_{1s} + (\overline{D}_1 - D_1)}{C_{1s} - \Sigma \Delta D_1} \times \frac{1}{\Delta t} = \frac{2 + (2 - 6)}{37.5 - (-1.0)} \times \frac{1}{1 \text{ yr}} = -0.052 \text{ per PY}$$

$$B_1 = R_{1b} - R_1 = -.052 - .053 = -0.105 \text{ per PY}$$

$$l_1 = C_{1.} - \overline{C}_1 - \Sigma \Delta D_1 = 45.4 - 30.3 - (-1.0) = 16.1$$

$$R_{1bl} = \frac{D_{1s} + (\overline{D}_1 - D_{1.})}{C_{1s} - (C_{1.} - \overline{C}_1)} \times \frac{1}{\Delta t} = \frac{2 + (2 - 6)}{37.5 - (45.4 - 30.3)} \times \frac{1}{1 \text{ yr}} = -0.089 \text{ per PY}$$

$$LT_1 = R_{1bl} - R_{1b} = -0.089 - (0.052) = -0.037 \text{ per PY}$$

---

screening examinations, these results do not pertain to specific years of follow-up after diagnosis but are averages for the program as a whole [expression (6–6)]. Except for the first year, the rates with the benefit of early treatment removed (R_{ib}) were greater than the crude rates, as would be expected. The negative reduction in case fatality from early treatment in the first year corresponds to the fact that D_0 is greater than $\overline{D}_0$, that is, more breast cancer deaths occurred in the screened group than in the control group. The greatest reduction in case fatality from early treatment occurred in the fourth through sixth years after entry. This was the period in which there was the greatest difference in the number of breast cancer deaths between the groups.

As a result of lead time, R_{ibl} is greater than R_{ib} for the second through sixth years of the program. In the first year, R_{ibl} is less than R_{ib} as a result of the negative value of R_{ib}. In the seventh year, R_{ibl} is slightly less than R_{ib} as a result of the negative value of l_i for that year. These negative values were, presumably, chance occurrences.

Table 6–3a also gives the case-fatality among prevalent cases in the control group according to year after entry irrespective of time of diagnosis. Thus, the value for each year corresponds to $E\{R_T\}$ as given by expression (6–7). In the first two years of the program, the CFR of screen-detected cases with benefit and lead time removed (R_{ibl}) was less than $E\{R_i\}$, the CFR in the control group. For each of the next five years, R_{ibl} was greater than $E\{R_i\}$. Over the first seven years, the average value of R_{ibl} was 0.101, slightly *higher* than the average value of $E\{R_i\}$, 0.098. Therefore, there is no evidence that screen-detected breast cancers progressed relatively slowly after the effect of early treatment is taken into account.

As with analyses of the lead time created by screening (chapter 3) and the effect of early treatment on mortality (chapter 4), analyses of the CFR could be done for subsets of study subjects, provided that such groups are not defined in ways that depend on the diagnostic effects of screening. For example, analyses of the CFR in the HIP study could be done according to age at entry or certain histologic characteristics such as degree of malignancy (but not according to age at detection or stage at diagnosis). The results would bear on the natural history of breast cancer identified by screening done at different ages, or the natural history of screen-detected breast cancer with different histologic features.

LENGTH-BIASED SAMPLING: Some biological and mathematical considerations imply that disease detected by screening may progress at a different rate during the preclinical phase (and, perhaps, during the clinical phase as well) than disease that first comes to attention as a result of symptoms.

Hutchison and Shapiro (1968) pointed out that the average duration of the preclinical phase of screen-detected cases (including lead time) tends to be longer than the mean duration of the preclinical phase of routinely diagnosed cases. This difference arises because the probability that a given case is detected in the preclinical phase depends on its length. A case with a very short preclinical phase has little chance of being detected before it becomes clinical; a case with a preclinical phase many years long is very likely to be detected if screening is done. A tendency for screening to identify cases with a relatively long preclinical phase has been termed *length-biased sampling* (Zelen, 1976). The existence of a bias, however, is simply a matter of viewpoint. Screening involves a different method of identifying cases than clinical diagnosis does. The mean duration of the preclinical phase of screen-detected disease is "biased" only by comparison with routinely diagnosed disease.

Figure 3–6 indicates the relationship between the duration of the preclinical phase and the probability of detection in a screening program. Half of the incident cases that develop are shown to have a preclinical phase of one year; the other half, four years. With a single screening examination, the probability of detection is four times as great for a case with a preclinical phase of four years as for a case with a preclinical phase of one year. Therefore, four "long" cases will be detected for every "short" case, if the incidences of long and short cases are equal.

If the preclinical phase of the disease can be divided into a nondetectable period and a uniformly detectable preclinical phase (UDPP) (see chapter 3), the extent of length-biased sampling can be defined as the difference of the average duration of the UDPP in screen-detected cases and its average duration in all cases that come to medical attention, whether or not detection occurred by screening. Given a steady state, the mean duration of the UDPP of *all* cases can be estimated from the prevalence of preclinical disease as detected at the initial screen, and the incidence rate of the disease: $\bar{d}_p \doteq P/I_c$ (expression (3–8)). The mean duration of the UDPP of *screen-detected* cases is twice their mean lead time. Thus, the extent of length-biased sampling (*LB*) is

$$LB = (2 \times \bar{L}) - \bar{d}_p \qquad (6–8)$$

Length-biased sampling is likely to be the greatest for cases detected at the initial screen, when the prevalent pool of preclinical cases is heavily weighted by those with long preclinical phases. As screening examinations are repeated, especially at short intervals, the distribution of durations of the preclinical phase among screen-detected cases more closely resembles that for routinely diagnosed disease in an unscreened population, and there would be less length bias.

It seems possible that cases progressing slowly (or rapidly) when preclinical continue to do the same when clinical. In other words, the length of the preclinical phase of disease is correlated with the length of the clinical phase. If this is so, screening would tend to detect cases destined to have a favorable prognosis (low CFR, long survival), regardless of lead time or any benefit of early treatment, as a result of length-biased sampling (Zelen, 1976). This is one mechanism that might lead to positive prognostic selection (expression (6–5)). There may be features of a disease that can shed light on this possibility. For example, histologic grade—the relative degree of histologic malignancy of a cancer—is believed to be related to its growth rate and is a predictor of the prognosis of the disease. The distribution of histologic grade could be compared between screen-detected and routinely diagnosed disease. Provided that the histologic grade is constant with time, more favorable grades among screen-detected cases would support the idea that slowly growing disease is identified preferentially. Anderson et al (1986) reported that the histologic types of breast cancers detected at the first screen of a series implied a probability of survival that was higher than that implied by the histologic types of cancers detected at later screens. Comparisons of stage distribution are likely to be misleading in this regard because lead time, as well as growth rate, determine stage at diagnosis.

Note that the lengths of the clinical phases of the *total* group of cases, screen-detected or not, that are diagnosed in the course of a program, are not affected by length-biased sampling. Screening changes the time of diagnosis but not the underlying biologic features of the disease. Length-biased sampling implies only that cases destined to have a slow or rapid clinical course preferentially come to attention through screening. Length-biased sampling is not the same process as the identification of pseudo-disease. The latter is disease with indefinite lead time but no implication as to what the prognosis would be after diagnosis as a result of symptoms.

Pseudodisease affects the average length of the preclinical phase of screen-detected disease, but the effect of all lead time, including that from pseudodisease, is removed in expression (6–3). Therefore, length-biased sampling and other types of prognostic selection—expression (6–5)—pertain only to events that occur after the lead time.

As described above, length-biased sampling is based on a very simple concept of the preclinical natural history: At some point in its development, a disease becomes readily detectable and remains so. However, a disease may not pass through a clearly defined UDPP. Instead, detectability might increase gradually as the time approaches at which symptoms would appear. In this situation, the average duration of the preclinical phase has no operational meaning, and it cannot be assumed that cases are identified on average, at its midpoint. Therefore, expression (6–8) would not correctly indicate the extent of length-biased sampling. Screen-detected cases would still be expected to have preclinical disease for a longer time than would routinely diagnosed cases. However, it would be necessary to know the patterns of detectability, or sensitivity functions (chapter 3), of individual cases to determine how great this difference is. The discussion also assumed that the *detectability* of a case during the preclinical phase is not related to its length. A comparatively high proportion of cases with long preclinical phases would be detected only because such cases are in the preclinical phase, at risk of being detected, for longer periods. The problems of length-biased sampling and its relation to prognosis become more complex if this condition is not met.

Suppose that detectability at screening tends to be greater for cases with relatively *short* preclinical phases. This would be true for a test based on exfoliative cytology, if faster-growing cases, with shorter preclinical phases, are more likely to shed abnormal cells. If such a disease has a clearly defined UDPP, the extent of length-biased sampling as measured by expression (6–8) would be less than that for a disease in which detection is related solely to the length of the preclinical phase. That is, the tendency of screening to identify cases with long preclinical phases would be counterbalanced to some degree by the fact that the most readily detectable cases are progressing quickly and, thus, have relatively short preclinical phases. Furthermore, the prognosis of screen-detected cases might not be comparatively favorable, since detected cases would tend to be progressing relatively fast. This possibility is illustrated well by results obtained from cytologic testing for cancer of the bladder in urologic outpatients. Farrow (1979) reported that bladder cancer that was positive by urinary cytology appeared much more malignant histologically than did cytologically negative cases diagnosed by other means. These data are shown in Table 6–4. The frequency of grade 3–4 tumors (most malignant appearance) was

Table 6–4. Percentage Distribution of Histologic Grade of Bladder Cancer According to Result of Urine Cytology

Histologic grade	Result of cytology		
	Positive	Atypical	Negative
1	5.4%	15.3%	42.2%
2	44.1	51.4	48.1
3	44.4	30.6	7.8
4	6.1	2.8	1.9
(N)	(408)	(72)	(154)

Source: Farrow GM: Pathologist's role in bladder cancer. *Semin Oncol* 1978; 6:198–206. Reprinted by permission of Grune & Stratton, Inc.

50.5% among patients with positive cytology but only 9.7% among those with negative cytology. Since histologic appearance generally is correlated with prognosis, this result is the reverse of what would be expected on the basis of length-biased sampling alone; cytologic detection of bladder cancer has brought more malignant, rather than less malignant, cases to attention.

The small amount of information available on the clinical course of screen-detected bladder cancer also suggests that cytologic testing leads to the detection of relatively malignant cases. Shaw (1977) reported figures on the survival of patients with bladder cancer detected by screening *v* the survival of patients that were not found by screening. Although the numbers of subjects were small, the results suggested longer survival for cases *not* detected by screening. Observed differences in the survival of screen-detected *v* routinely diagnosed bladder cancer may even understate the degree to which cytologic screening leads to the detection of relatively malignant cases; adjustment for lead time would increase the prognostic difference in favor of the routinely diagnosed cases. Moreover, it is possible that the screen-detected cases benefited from early treatment. Had the screen-detected cases not been treated early, their prognosis could have been even poorer. Cartwright et al (1981) also reported on survival in cytology-detected *v* routinely diagnosed bladder cancer. They found that survival tended to be somewhat greater in the screen-detected series. The screen-detected group, however, had been screened very intensively—monthly—and no interval cases were found. The very frequent screening may have eliminated prognostic selection and maximized the lead time.

In short, screening might select cases that are either favorable or unfavorable prognostically. If screening detects cases with relatively long preclinical phases, their prognosis would be relatively good; if cases with relatively short preclinical phases are detected, their prognosis would be relatively poor, assuming a positive correlation of the lengths of the preclinical and clinical phases. These possibilities are not mutually exclusive. In bladder cancer, it appears that cytologic screening may detect unfavorable cases. Among cases with a given degree of detectability, however, it could be that the cases detected by screening would include a disproportionate number with longer preclinical phases and, perhaps, longer clinical phases.

The possibility of "reverse" length-biased sampling underscores two important points. First, observed case fatality is not a valid measure of the efficacy of screening and early treatment. Use of this measure might suggest that persons with screen-detected bladder cancer are actually harmed. In fact, the efficacy of screening and early treatment in bladder cancer has not yet been evaluated, and it is conceivable that early treatment of prognostically unfavorable cases would lengthen their lives. Second, the difference in the average length of the preclinical phase between screen-detected and routinely diagnosed disease is determined by variability in the detectability of the disease as well as by variability in its rate of progression.

The distribution of lead time derived from a statistical model (chapter 3) may be used to remove the effect of lead time from the CFR of screen-detected cases. Walter and Stitt (1987) assumed that lead time in breast screening follows a negative exponential distribution as suggested by Walter and Day (1983). The ten-year cumulative case fatality (CCF) in screen-detected cases, with correction for the lead time, is 39% lower than the CCF in the control group. The reduction in breast cancer deaths attributable to early treatment was estimated as 20.7 by comparison with interval cases and as 19.2 by comparison with women who refused screening. Walter and Stitt also fitted the HIP data with a more complex model that allowed for a correlation of lead time and the CFR during the clinical phase. There was only a slight difference in the predicted benefit of screening by use of this model v the simpler one. The fitted values, however, did indicate a correlation between the lead time and the subsequent CFR. The length of the preclinical phase could not be distinguished from the amount of lead time because the length of the preclinical phase is assumed to follow a negative exponential distribution. As Walter and Stitt (1987) note, however, long lead times can only occur in cases with long preclinical phases. Thus, their findings imply a relation between the length of the preclinical phase and the CFR after the lead time. Length bias is an explanation of this relationship, but it is not the only one. Treatment might be effective for cases with moderate or long lead times but ineffective for cases with short lead times. The effect of treatment, as well as that of lead time, should be removed from the CFR in order to investigate prognostic selection bias.

Models to analyze the CFR provide a nonexperimental approach to evaluating the effect of screening on mortality. An advantage of this approach is that it can be based on data from screened subjects only (Walter and Stitt, 1987). This feature might be useful when suitable unscreened comparison subjects either do not exist or cannot be identified. Otherwise, evaluation by use of such models offers no advantages over the basic nonexperimental follow-up or case-control methods. The analysis by models cannot be done earlier than the other methods can because they all require observations of deaths among screen-detected cases. Furthermore, data on the incidence of the disease among unscreened subjects, if available, should be included in an analysis by models (Walter and Day, 1983). Finally, the validity of some components of the model may be questionable; use of an incorrect model could create misleading results.

7 The Feasibility of Screening Programs

From a practical perspective, screening compares unfavorably with other means of disease control such as avoidance of environmental hazards and immunization. A screening examination can only help people who already have preclinical disease, so screening generally must be repetitive to maintain a useful level of disease control, and the resulting high costs are a serious obstacle. Moreover, adverse effects, especially false-positive results, are relatively common.

A number of conditions must be met for the advantages of screening to outweigh the disadvantages. Obviously, the test used should be relatively inexpensive, convenient and painless, and safe. Given such a test, a screening program must be organized to function effectively and economically. In a cervical cytology program, for example (Task Force, 1976), attention must be given to:

Initial training and continuing education of professional and technical personnel
Organization of individual screening and laboratory facilities
Coordination of screening facilities
Coordination of laboratory facilities
Relation to screening programs for other diseases
Encouraging participation of the target population
Obtaining specimens
Transporting specimens
Methods of laboratory analysis
Quality control
Interpretation of test results
Reporting test results to screening facilities and screenees
Diagnostic follow-up of positive tests

Operational issues of these types are not discussed here, but their importance is great. A screening program may succeed or fail depending on the choices that are made intentionally or by default. A question that is likely to arise in the course of creating a populationwide program of mammographic screening for breast cancer is whether the program should be carried on by departments of general diagnostic radiology, or by new specialized units. The best approach is not obvious. The start-up costs certainly would be lower with a program based in existing organizations. Given a connection with established patterns of medical care, such a program might be relatively successful at attracting participants. On the other hand, the cost per examination might be too high. Intermingling the screening mammograms with diagnostic studies could have an adverse effect on the quality of screening, especially its specificity. Moreover, the quality of screening as practiced in the community may not be as high as that in specialized programs (McClatchey et al, 1989).

However a program is operated, the frequency of true-positive cases detected must be reasonably high, and the frequency of false-positive tests relatively low. If the frequency of case detection is low, there will not be sufficient return for the costs of screening. False positives lead to the additional costs and other adverse effects of diagnostic examinations from which the patients derive no benefit. The frequencies of true positives and false positives depend on test characteristics—sensitivity and specificity—on the screening schedule, and on the prevalence of preclinical disease in the target population. This chapter describes these relationships and shows how they can be manipulated to improve the feasibility of screening programs. Factors that contribute to high costs are described, and possible ways of reducing them are indicated.

TRUE POSITIVES

The success of screening at identifying cases of preclinical disease is usually described as the proportion of screened subjects found to have the disease, that is, the detected prevalence. Table 7–1 presents the results of the initial screening examination for the first 20,211 women screened in the HIP program. Of this number, 55 women were found to have breast cancer. Thus, the detected prevalence was 2.7 per 1,000 women screened. The detected prevalence of disease depends on the sensitivity function of the test used, and the distribution of potential lead times. According to the notation given in chapters 3 and 6, s_j is the sensitivity of the test for cases with potential lead time j; k_j is the number of such cases tested; N_0 is the

Table 7–1. Results of Initial Screening Examination in the HIP Program

Result	Number
Recommendation for biopsy or aspiration	510
Biopsy performed	307
Pathologically confirmed breast cancer	55
No recommendation for biopsy	19,701
Total screened	20,211
Total not found to have breast cancer	20,156

Source: Shapiro et al (1967).

total number of persons (cases plus noncases) tested; and C_{0s} is the number of cases detected. The detected prevalence can be written as

$$\frac{\sum_j s_j k_j}{N_0} = \frac{C_{0s}}{N_0}$$

The total number of preclinical cases tested is $\sum_j k_j$. If this number were known, an estimate of the average sensitivity of the test would be $C_{0s}/\sum_j k_j$. Therefore, the prevalence of detected cases can be thought of as

$$\frac{\text{Average sensitivity} \times \text{Number of preclinical cases}}{\text{Number of persons tested}}$$

An example is given with artificial data in Table 7–2, part A. At the time of screening the number of cases of preclinical breast cancer is $a + c = 500$. The average sensitivity of the test $= a/(a + c) = 80\%$. There were 100,000 people tested. Therefore, the prevalence of detected cases is

$$\frac{[a/(a + c)] \times (a + c)}{100,000} = \frac{a}{100,000} = \frac{400}{100,000}$$

The detected prevalence could be raised by improving the sensitivity characteristics of the test. The detected prevalence also would be higher if the test were applied to a population in which the true prevalence of preclinical disease is higher.

FALSE POSITIVES

A *false positive* is a screened person with a positive test who is found, on diagnostic evaluation, not to have the disease of interest. A false positive may be the result of a test error or of the presence of the sign on which

Table 7–2. Hypothetical Data Related to Initial Screening of 100,000 Women for Breast Cancer

Test outcomes	Preclinical breast cancer					
	A. Yes	No	Total	B. Yes	No	Total
Positive	400 (a)	995 (b)	1,395 (a + b)	400 (a)	1,990 (b)	2,390 (a + b)
Negative	100 (c)	98,505 (d)	98,605 (c + d)	100 (c)	97,510 (d)	97,610 (c + d)
Total	500 (a + c)	99,500 (b + d)	100,000 (N)	500 (a + c)	99,500 (b + d)	100,000 (N)

Source: Cole and Morrison (1980).

Average sensitivity	$\dfrac{a}{a + c}$	A. $\dfrac{400}{500} = 80\%$	B. $\dfrac{400}{500} = 80\%$
Specificity	$\dfrac{d}{b + d}$	$\dfrac{98,505}{99,500} = 99\%$	$\dfrac{97,510}{99,500} = 98\%$
Predictive value	$\dfrac{a}{a + b}$	$\dfrac{400}{1,395} = 29\%$	$\dfrac{400}{2,390} = 17\%$

the test is based in someone who does not have the disease. False positives may be divided into two groups: those not found to have any disease, and those found to have some other disease. The latter group may be at elevated risk for the target condition and deserve special attention for that reason. For example, a cause of false positives in breast cancer screening is benign breast neoplasia, which is a precursor of breast cancer (Kelsey, 1979; Kelsey and Gamman, 1990). The significance of false positives without any apparent disease is not known. Patients with pseudodisease could be thought of as being yet a third group of false positives. Individual patients with pseudodisease cannot, however, be distinguished from true positives.

The frequency of false positives at a given screen is determined primarily by the specificity of the test used. Since preclinical cases cannot be false positives, the prevalence of preclinical disease is another determinant of the number of false positives in a group that is screened, but the prevalence of preclinical disease in an asymptomatic population will usually be so low that its effect on false positives is of no importance.

SPECIFICITY

The specificity of a test is defined as the proportion of screened persons without preclinical disease who are designated correctly as negative.

$$\text{Specificity} = \frac{\text{Number negative on test}}{\text{Total number tested who do not have preclinical disease}}$$

(7-1)

The number of nondiseased persons found to be negative is equal to the number of nondiseased persons tested minus the number of false positives. As with sensitivity, a value of specificity probably should be viewed as referring to particular circumstances, since the probability that a test is positive in people without the disease depends on their physiologic characteristics and the prevalence of other diseases—factors that are likely to vary.

In principle, the definition of specificity is beset by some of the difficulties with the definition of sensitivity given by expression (3-1). Knowledge of the number in the denominator of expression (7-1) requires the application of a diagnostic test, which may itself be in error. In addition, there are many diseases for which diagnostic tests are expensive, uncomfortable, or risky, and therefore would not be done on asymptomatic people with negative screening tests. Most diseases for which screening is done are sufficiently uncommon, however, for a satisfactory estimate of specificity to be obtained by taking as nondiseased everyone not found to have the disease in the course of a screening program. The latter group includes persons truly nondiseased, as well as false negatives—diseased people with negative screening tests—but if the disease is uncommon, the proportion of diseased people included would be very small.

Refer again to Table 7–2, part A. The denominator of the specificity should be 99,500, the number of nondiseased women. In practice, this number would not be known unless everyone had diagnostic studies. However, the number of women not found to have breast cancer (100,000 − 400 = 99,600) differs from the correct denominator by only the 100 women who were false negatives. Similarly the correct numerator (98,505) would not be known, but it is approximated well by the number that tested negative (98,605). The specificity could then be estimated as 98,605/99,600 = 99.001%, which is virtually equal to the correct value, 98,505/99,500 = 99.000%. (A simpler—although less accurate—approximation is the prevalence of negative tests, 98.605%.)

The specificity of screening for breast cancer by mammography and physical examination may be estimated with data from the HIP program (Table 7–1). If a *recommendation* for biopsy is taken as a positive screening examination, the specificity would be approximated, as outlined above, as (20,211 − 510)/20,156 = 98%. If the *performance* of a biopsy is taken as an indicator of a positive test, the specificity would be (20,211 − 307)/20,156 = 99%.

During the planning phase of a screening program, it is important to obtain a preliminary estimate of the specificity of the screening procedure to be used in order to ensure that the program will not be swamped with false positives. As indicated in chapter 3, preliminary information on the characteristics of a screening test sometimes can be obtained in the course of differential diagnosis. Refer again to Table 3–1, which gives data on the use of urine cytology for the diagnosis of bladder cancer. Among 8,916 patients found to be free of cancer, the cytology result was "malignant" in 92 and "atypical" in 228. If only patients with malignant cytology are considered positive, the specificity is estimated as (8,586 + 228)/8,916 = 99%. If atypical cytology also is considered positive, the specificity would be 8,596/8,916 = 96%. Either estimate would tend to be less than the corresponding specificity in screening asymptomatic people, if people without cancer who attend an outpatient clinic are more likely than are asymptomatic people to have some condition that would lead to a positive test. Provided that the estimate is reasonably good, however, the proportion expected to have false-positive tests in a screening program would be approximately equal to one minus the specificity of the test, or the nonspecificity.

PREDICTIVE VALUE

The predictive value (PV) is the proportion of people with a positive screening test who are found by diagnostic evaluation to have the disease in question (Vecchio, 1966). In Table 7–2, part A, the PV is $a/(a + b) =$ 29%. In the HIP program (Table 7–1), the PV was $55/510 = 11\%$ if a recommendation for biopsy is taken as a positive screen, and $55/307 =$ 18% if the performance of a biopsy is taken as positive. Both the PV of a screening program and the specificity of a screening test are negatively related to the frequency of false positives. The PV is equal to one minus the proportion of false positives among positive screenees. The specificity is equal to one minus the proportion of false positives among nondiseased people tested. Each of these proportions has been referred to as the "false positive rate." This term should be abandoned because of its ambiguity.

The components of the PV of a given screening examination in a program are the number of true positive cases detected and the number of false positives. Thus, a high PV is the result of conditions that lead to a relatively high number of detected cases (high prevalence of preclinical disease and a test with good sensitivity characteristics) and a relatively low number of false positives (high test specificity). The usefulness of the PV is limited by the fact that it is a proportional measure. The same PV could be observed in a screening program with a very high, or very low, frequency of detected cases, with corresponding implications for disease control.

A small change in test specificity may have a large effect on the PV. Suppose the results in Table 7–2, part A were changed to reflect a specificity of 98%, rather than 99%, leading to the numbers in Table 7–2, part B. In this case, the PV would be $400/(400 + 1990) = 17\%$. To bring about the same decrease in PV, the average sensitivity would have to fall from 80% to 40%. The PV is affected equally by proportionally equivalent but inverse changes in the sensitivity and the *non*specificity.

The significance of a low PV depends very much on the consequences of a positive test. If it is followed simply by a repetition of the screening test as in screening for hypertension, or some other inexpensive and innocuous procedure, then a low PV might well be acceptable. If, however, a positive screening test is followed by an expensive or potentially harmful diagnostic examination (as for cancer of the colon) then it is important to achieve a high PV. A poor PV may also lead to lack of acceptance of a screening program by the target population because of a widespread perception that a positive screening test is likely to be a false alarm.

ENHANCEMENT OF THE FEASIBILITY OF SCREENING PROGRAMS

Attempts may be made to (1) increase the number of cases detected, (2) decrease the number of false positives, and (3) screen only a high-risk segment of the population in order to detect most of the cases that would be detected by screening the entire population, but reduce the overall cost of screening and the number of false positives.

The number of cases detected can be increased in several ways. The simplest is to lower the criterion of positivity. The criterion is the point that divides positive from negative test results. A change in the criterion affects both the sensitivity and specificity of the test.

Some tests, such as that for intraocular pressure, have continuous outcomes. Other tests have "yes or no" outcomes; sigmoidoscopy is an example. Although there is no stated numerical criterion of positivity, there is, nonetheless, an implicit criterion: the degree of mucosal abnormality that the examiner believes to warrant a biopsy or other studies.

Suppose that a population is tested for intraocular pressure in order to detect asymptomatic glaucoma. Figure 7–1 shows the distributions of test results that might be obtained, and a criterion of positivity.[1] As is typical in screening, there is a large number of people without disease and a small number with. These groups have generally different test outcomes. People with glaucoma tend to have relatively high intraocular pressure, compared to unaffected people. However, there is some overlap of results in diseased and nondiseased people. Either because of test error or physiologic variation, a measurement of intraocular pressure may be unusually high in someone without the disease, or unusually low in someone with it. If the criterion of positivity were taken to be 25 mm, as shown, people with glaucoma who have this value or higher when tested would be true positives. Diseased subjects with a test result lower than 25 mm would have their status designated incorrectly; they are false negatives. The average sensitivity would be the stippled area (true positives) divided by the total area enclosed by distribution B (true positives plus false negatives). The specificity would be the cross-hatched area (true negatives) divided by the total area of distribution A (true negatives plus false positives). The PV would be the stippled area (true positives) divided by the sum of the stippled area plus the plain portion of distribution A (true positives plus false positives).

If the criterion of positivity is lowered, a less extreme test result (eg, a lower intraocular pressure) is considered to be positive and a higher pro-

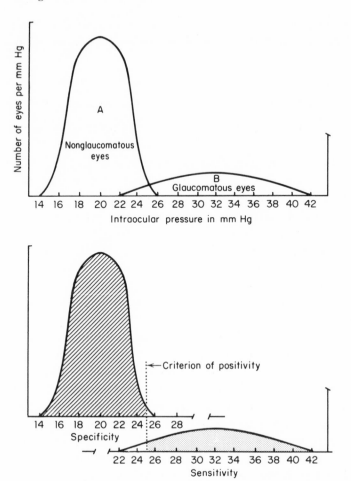

Figure 7–1. Relationship of sensitivity and specificity to distribution of test results and criterion of positivity.

Source: Thorner and Remein (1967).

portion of diseased people are detected. That is, the average sensitivity of the test increases. But, because of the overlap of test results between diseased and nondiseased people, the proportion of positives among the nondiseased—false positives—increases, and the specificity of the test decreases. Because the number of nondiseased people greatly exceeds the number of diseased, even a small decrease in specificity may lead to a very large increase in the number of false positives and a large decrease in the PV.

Table 7–3 gives the sensitivity, specificity, and PV based on the urine cytology results in outpatients (Table 3–1), for two criteria of positivity:

Table 7-3. Sensitivity, Specificity, and Predictive Value in Cytologic Screening for Bladder Cancer, According to Criterion of Positivity (based on Table 3-1)

Criterion	Sensitivity (%)	Specificity (%)	Predictive value (%)
Malignant	53	99	82
Atypical	67	96	73

Source: Farrow GM: Pathologist's role in bladder cancer. *Semin Oncol* 1978; 6:198–206. Reprinted by permission of Grune & Stratton, Inc.

malignant and atypical. The lower criterion, atypical, yields a higher sensitivity, but lower specificity and lower PV, than the higher criterion does. (Note that the two indicators of a positive test in the HIP—recommendation of biopsy and its performance—are not simple adjustments of the criterion of positivity. A recommendation not followed by a biopsy does not lead to either a confirmed diagnosis or a false positive.)

In addition to lowering the criterion of positivity, the number of cases detected can be increased by increasing the frequency of screening, or by using two or more different tests and considering a positive result on any one as an indication for a diagnostic examination (Frankenburg, 1975). In each instance, a person with preclinical disease is more likely to be detected because more tests are done. For the same reason, someone without disease is more likely to test positive and to require diagnostic studies. Prenatal screening for Down syndrome, for example, can be done simply in relation to maternal age. Women whose age is at least as high as the criterion value are offered a diagnostic test (karyotype of fetal cells in amniotic fluid). If the criterion of positivity is age 38, the sensitivity of testing is estimated to be 20%; about 20% of all cases of Down syndrome occur in pregnancies with maternal age at least 38. The specificity of this procedure is 97.9%; 2.1% of unaffected pregnancies occur at age 38 or above (Cuckle et al, 1984).

Another screening test for Down syndrome is the level of AFP in maternal serum. Relatively low values are associated with the disease. By use of the AFP test with a criterion of positivity of 0.5 times the median value in normal pregnancies, the sensitivity would be 21% and the specificity, 95%. The sensitivity can be increased by using both the AFP test and maternal age to identify women to be offered a diagnostic test. A woman could be considered to test positive if her expected age at delivery is at least 38 *or* her AFP test is equal to or less than 0.5 times the median. The sensitivity of this procedure is 36% and the specificity is 93%.

The use of multiple tests, or of more frequent screening, has the effect of lowering the criterion of positivity; the numbers of both true positives and false positives will increase. The total costs and the cost per detected case also will increase. It is a matter of judgment as to whether the trade-off is worthwhile in a given setting. Frequent screening lowers the subsequent prevalence of preclinical disease. Therefore, continued frequent screening may lead to very unfavorable feasibility characteristics: a low prevalence of detected cases and a poor PV for the program as a whole.

The numbers of false positives can be decreased by means opposite to those that increase the numbers of true positives. First, the criterion of positivity can be raised. The feasibility of a screening program may be more readily improved by raising than by lowering the criterion. Because the number of nondiseased people far exceeds the number of diseased people, raising the criterion slightly can greatly reduce the number of false positives at the cost of losing only a small number of true positives. A similar effect might be achieved by decreasing the frequency of screening, or by screening with a series of tests and taking as positive only screenees with a positive result on all tests. For example, diagnostic testing for Down syndrome could be offered only to women who are at least a given age (eg, 38 years) *and* whose AFP value falls at or below the median value. Seventy-nine percent of cases of Down syndrome and 46% of unaffected pregnancies had AFP levels at or below the median value (Cuckle et al, 1984). Compared to screening based on maternal age alone, therefore, the two tests together would identify about four-fifths as many cases of Down syndrome and create about half as many false positives, assuming independence of the tests. It would also be possible to rescreen initial positives with the same test and take only the second result as the outcome of screening (Cuckle and Wald, 1984).

In some circumstances, a variable criterion of positivity may be used to balance the benefits *v* adverse effects and costs of screening. For example, the level of maternal AFP taken to be positive in screening for Down syndrome could increase with maternal age. A woman could be considered to test positive if her expected age at delivery is at least 38 years or, if 25 to 38 years, the AFP is equal to or less than a cut-off that increases with increasing age from 0.5 to 1.0 times the median. This procedure has a sensitivity of 40% and a specificity of 93.2% (Cuckle et al, 1984). The sensitivity is higher, and the specificity the same, as in screening with a fixed criterion of positivity for AFP. This approach exploits the increasing prevalence of Down syndrome with increasing maternal age.

It may be possible to increase the sensitivity or the specificity (or both) without loss to the other by means of technical improvements in the screening procedure. However, this goal might be difficult to achieve and yet have the test remain sufficiently convenient and inexpensive. In some circumstances, tests with numerical outcomes might be repeated and the measurements averaged before referring to the criterion of positivity. The resulting reduction in random variation could improve both the sensitivity and the specificity.

It is always worth considering a number of approaches to improving the operation of a screening program, since some approaches may work, and others not, in particular circumstances. Suppose, for example, that a program is threatened by excessive numbers of false positives. In a screening program for glaucoma, the problem might be solved by making a minor upward adjustment in the criterion of positivity. However, this situation might not be practical in a program directed at cervical cancer. Fine gradations in the degree of malignancy in cytologic specimens are difficult to recognize reliably, and it may not be possible to make a small, carefully calibrated change in the criterion of positivity. Furthermore, a large increase in the criterion could lead to an unacceptable decrease in case finding. Repeated testing would be uneconomical, and, in any event, would fail to eliminate biologic false positives—positive tests owing to benign abnormalities that cannot be distinguished from cancer. The best approach is likely to be an adjustment of the screening frequency. Since the preclinical phase of cervical cancer tends to be long, a moderate decrease in screening frequency, say from every year to every two or three years, would have only a slight adverse effect on case finding and on reduction in mortality (chapter 11), but there would be a dramatic decrease in false positives and other costs of screening.

HIGH-RISK GROUPS: If a disease is very rare, the cost of screening will probably be very high in relation to the gain. Because almost all the persons screened are not diseased, there will also be many false positives for each true positive—a low PV. A low PV in itself is undesirable, and diagnostic studies of the false positives increase the costs even further without commensurate benefits.

The feasibility of screening for a very rare disease can be enhanced by restricting the program to people among whom the prevalence of preclinical disease is high. The higher the prevalence, the greater the return for a given investment of resources, other things being equal. The prevalence of preclinical disease depends on its incidence rate and average duration. For most diseases there is presently little or no information about the way in which the duration of preclinical disease varies with its incidence. Therefore, the prevalence of preclinical disease often is assumed to be high in groups for which incidence or mortality rates are high. All screening involves the preliminary identification of groups at relatively high risk (the target population) according to age, sex, race, residence, etc. Information on additional risk indicators might be derived from specialized epidemiologic studies. The use of this information to designate high-risk groups is simply an extension of the process by which a target population is identified.

Screening tests and indicators of high risk are logically equivalent. As described above, maternal age at conception, a risk indicator for Down syndrome, may by itself serve as a screening test. The prevalence of pre-clinical disease among persons positive to an indicator of high risk is equivalent to the predictive value among persons with a positive screening test. The only reason to distinguish risk indicators from screening tests is one of feasibility and cost. Compared to screening, the assessment of risk indicators is easy, inexpensive, and free of medical hazard. The screening tests are done later in a sequence that identifies persons to be offered diagnostic testing.

A screened high-risk group realizes the benefits of the program while the costs of screening and of diagnostic procedures for false positives are kept relatively low. The population from which the high-risk group is selected suffers an overall reduction of benefit since low-risk people, among whom some disease occurs, are not screened at all. (If a disease occurs only in one sex or the other, the use of sex to identify the target population would entail no overall loss of benefit.) The balance of the saving in cost v the reduction of benefit to the entire population depends on the ability of a risk factor, or combination of factors, to select people who have the preclinical disease being screened for and a high ability to reject those who do not have it (Soini and Hakama, 1978). The first characteristic is the sensitivity of the risk factor and the second characteristic is its specificity.

If an indicator of high risk is not sensitive, a restricted program would not test a high proportion of people with the disease, and the overall decrease in mortality would be small. This loss of benefit to the general population may be of little concern when screening is used to alleviate a special problem in a setting of greatly elevated risk, such as an industry in which hazardous substances are handled.

Most diseases screened for are sufficiently uncommon for the specificity of the risk factor to be approximated by one minus the prevalence of the risk factor in the population. The less common an indicator of high risk is—the higher its specificity—the smaller the fraction of the total population that must be screened and the greater the savings in cost.

The issues related to high-risk groups are well illustrated by hypothetical mass screening for cancer of the bladder (Morrison, 1979b). As the disease is much more common in men than in women, research on screening for bladder cancer has concerned men primarily. Each year there are about 7,000 deaths from this disease among the 85 million U.S. men. Suppose that early diagnosis and treatment would reduce bladder cancer mortality by 50%, a figure that may be unrealistically high. If yearly screening were required to realize this gain, a program that would prevent 3,500 bladder cancer deaths annually would involve 85 million tests each year. Even if the specificity of the test were 99.9%, doing 85 million tests would result in 85,000 false positives requiring further evaluation.

Age is a relatively good indicator of high risk of bladder cancer. Eighty-seven percent of bladder cancer deaths in men occur in the 21% who are 60 years old or more. Screening only this age group in a program that reduces bladder cancer mortality by 50% would reduce bladder cancer mortality in *all* men by 43.5%. Further improvement in efficiency, with some loss of overall benefit, could be achieved by restricting screening to still older men, who have even higher rates. However, the use of age as a risk indicator for screening has an obvious drawback: Screening would be directed at finding those cases who have the least to gain in life expectancy.

In public health terms, cigarette smoking is the most important known cause of bladder cancer. Smokers have about twice the risk of nonsmokers, and about 50% of bladder cancer in men is attributable to cigarette smoking (IARC, 1986). Furthermore, about 85% of deaths from bladder cancer occur among men who have smoked. Thus it appears that a history of smoking is a fairly sensitive risk indicator.[2] However, smoking is common and not very specific to people with rare diseases such as bladder cancer; most people who smoke never develop bladder cancer.

Suppose that a screening program for bladder cancer in men were restricted to those with a history of smoking. Eighty-five percent of the potential bladder cancer deaths in the target population (eg, men 60 years of age and older) would be included in the screening program, so 85% of the total possible benefit would be realized. As a result, the population would experience a 50% × 85% = 42.5% reduction in bladder cancer mortality, as opposed to 50% if the entire population were screened. If, however, 73% of the men had smoked, as Cole (1973) found, then 73% of the target population would have to be screened to achieve 85% of the total possible benefit; the gain in efficiency is small and the costs would still be high (Table 7–4).

Bladder cancer risk is elevated in a number of occupations that are uncommon exposures compared to smoking (Silverman et al, 1992). Cole (1973) found that the relative risk was 1.8 in men employed in any of five hazardous occupations. About 25% of men were so exposed, but consider the very optimistic assumption that an occupational history would make it possible to identify the 1% of men among whom would occur all bladder cancer attributable to the five occupations. Nineteen percent of all bladder cancer deaths would occur in such a group (Table 7–4). In other words,

Table 7-4. Overall Reduction in Bladder Cancer Mortality in Men as a Result of Hypothetical Screening Programs Restricted to Cigarette Smokers or to Workers in Hazardous Occupations

Risk factor	Relative mortality[a]	Proportion exposed to factor[b]	Proportion of bladder cancer deaths among those with factor	Overall reduction in bladder cancer mortality from program that reduces mortality among the screened by 50%
Smoking	1.9	0.73	0.85	42.5%
Occupation	20.0	0.01	0.19	9.5%

Source: Morrison AS: Public health value of using epidemiologic information to identify high-risk groups for bladder cancer screening. *Semin Oncol* 1979; 6:184–188. Reprinted by permission of Grune & Stratton, Inc.

[a]Mortality rate for persons exposed relative to a rate of 1 for those not exposed.

[b]See test for definition of exposure.

this hypothetical history is quite specific, but not very sensitive. A screening program restricted to this group would be economical; 850,000 men would be screened instead of 85 million. However, only about 20% of the total possible gain would be achieved; the entire population of men would experience a 10%, rather than a 50%, reduction in bladder cancer mortality. The public health value of such a program would be small, although the gain to the men with a hazardous occupation would be substantial. In contrast, large proportions of deaths from pleural and peritoneal mesothelioma are attributable to occupational exposure to asbestos (Fraumeni and Blot, 1982). If good screening tests and effective early treatment for mesothelioma were available, screening based on occupation would have a relatively large impact on the overall rate.

Soini and Hakama (1978) investigated the use of combinations of epidemiologic risk factors in selecting high-risk groups in screening for breast cancer. They encountered conditions similar to those illustrated by the use of smoking history as a selective factor in bladder cancer screening: Although the risk indicators were reasonably sensitive, the high-risk group encompassed a large fraction of the total population. About two-thirds of the women were considered to be at high risk, and this segment included about four-fifths of the cases, one-fifth remaining in the low-risk segment. In screening for cervical cancer, on the other hand, selecting high-risk groups with epidemiologic risk factors led to conditions more like those illustrated by the use of occupation as a risk factor: The defined high-risk group included 8% of the population and only 39% of the cases (Hakama et al, 1979).

High-risk and low-risk groups might also be identified by use of information derived from screening tests themselves. This possibility has received the most attention in the context of screening for cervical cancer and breast cancer. A Canadian Task Force (1976), for example, suggested that women initially considered to be at high risk for cervical cancer be placed in an intermediate-risk group after two negative Pap smears.

In addition to revealing tumors, mammograms show morphologic features of nonmalignant breast tissue. These features have most often been categorized according to the "parenchymal pattern" (Wolfe, 1976). Women with the P2 (severe prominent ducts) or DY (dysplasia) patterns are at elevated risk compared to women with the N1 (normal) or P1 (mild prominent ducts) patterns (Saftlas and Szklo, 1987). The estimated percentages of breast tissue showing radiologic nodular densities or homogeneous density are important components of the parenchymal pattern, and these features also are related to the risk of subsequent breast cancer. Table 7–5 shows the relative risks of breast cancer associated with the parenchymal pattern and various amounts of nodular densities. By use of parenchymal features, women at quite high risk can be identified. The relative risk has been estimated as 10 in women under 60 with at least 40% of the breast showing nodular densities if the densities had an average diameter of at least 4 mm (Brisson et al, 1982a).

Table 7–5. Percentage Distributions of Breast Cancer Cases and Controls, Aged 20 to 59 Years, and Relative Risk According to Parenchymal Pattern and the Estimated Percentage of the Breast Showing Nodular Densities

Mammographic feature	Cases (%)	Controls (%)	Relative risk
Parenchymal pattern			
N1	3.4	8.4	1.0[a]
P1	24.8	36.9	1.7
P2	49.0	34.9	4.2
DY	22.8	19.8	4.0
Percent of breast showing nodular densities			
0	8.3	17.0	1.0[a]
1–19	18.0	27.5	1.8
20–39	33.5	27.5	3.6
40–59	20.9	14.1	5.1
60+	19.4	14.0	5.4
Number of subjects	206	808	

Source: Brisson et al (1982a).
[a]Reference group.

Mammographic screening is expensive and may lead to large numbers of biopsies of benign disease. The idea that information on parenchymal features might be used to reduce the costs and risks to a population that carries out mammographic screening is, therefore, very attractive. Parenchymal characteristics as determined from the initial (negative) mammogram would be used to adjust subsequent screening. For example, rescreening might be done every three years for women with an N1 or P1 pattern v every year for women with a P2 or DY pattern. In a study of breast cancer screening in Malmo, Sweden, the parenchymal features at early examinations are used to determine whether later mammography is done by the one-view or two-view method (Andersson et al, 1988) (chapter 9). The design of that study will not, however, result in an estimate of the value of that procedure. The information is not yet available to devise a satisfactory and rational set of rescreening schedules based on mammographic features, for the following reasons.

1. The sensitivity or specificity of mammographic features as indicators of high risk is not satisfactory. Suppose that screening is limited to the group described above that has a relative risk of 10. This group constitutes about two percent of women under 60. The remaining women, however, would be at moderate to high risk, rather than low risk. It does not seem justified to exclude such women from a screening program. Instead, a larger group of women, those whose relative risk of breast cancer is at least 3.5, could be taken to be at high risk. This group might include about 55% of women (under 60 years of age) identified by either a P2 or DY parenchymal pattern, or 20% or more of the breast with nodular densities. Such a group would not be small enough to result in a large increase in efficiency, and there would still be an unacceptably high rate of breast cancer in the unscreened group.

2. Only a little is known about the relation of mammographic parenchymal features to breast cancer over a period of more than a few years (Brisson et al, 1988). Data on long-term relationships are essential in formulating screening policy, particularly in establishing rescreening intervals for women initially at low risk.

3. Distributions of parenchymal features appear to vary with age. Generally, the features change in a way that suggests lower risk with increasing age (Brisson et al, 1982b). Whether—and how—age-related changes modify the risk as inferred from an initial mammogram is not known.

4. Perhaps most important, the value of early treatment has not been related to a woman's apparent level of risk. The mammographic features indicative of risk are radiologic densities that may obscure tumors at screening, leading to differences in the characteristics of tumors detected

in high-risk v low-risk women. For a given frequency of screening, it is possible that tumors detected in high-risk women are relatively advanced and less amenable to treatment.

BENEFITS VERSUS ADVERSE EFFECTS—THE INDIVIDUAL'S PERSPECTIVE

A person who has a screening test for a chronic disease ultimately falls into one of the groups shown in Table 7–6. The group to which a given person belongs may not be known. For example, it is not possible to determine whether an individual death has been postponed, so that people who belong to group A_1 cannot be distinguished from those who belong to group A_2, and it may not be possible to distinguish true negatives (D) from false negatives (C). On the other hand, true positives (groups A_1 and A_2) are readily distinguished from false positives (group B).

Table 7–6 gives a rough indication of the relative value of each outcome to a participant in a screening program.

People in group A_1—true positives whose deaths are postponed by early treatment—obviously benefit as a result of screening. The gain in life outweighs any costs or other adverse effects of screening. However, this is the only group with a strongly favorable outcome.

It is uncertain as to whether people in groups A_2 and D gain or lose from screening. People in group A_2 learn of their disease earlier than they would otherwise, but they do not have their lives extended. It may be useful in planning one's affairs to learn of a serious disease early. However, an early diagnosis may have drawbacks. Patients might experience anxiety from awareness of their disease and morbidity as a result of treatment sooner than they otherwise would. Treatment might be relatively innocuous, but it might, on the other hand, cause a serious deterioration in the quality of life, as would a colostomy or a urine diversion procedure. A period of morbidity that is the result of screening and that is not compensated by gain in life probably should be considered an adverse effect. This is especially

Table 7–6. Relative Value of Various Outcomes of Screening

Group	Outcome	Value
A_1	True positive; death postponed	Large benefit
A_2	True positive; death not postponed	Questionable
B	False positive	Moderate adverse effect
C	False negative	Small adverse effect
D	True negative	Questionable

true for someone with pseudodisease who, in the usual course of events, would never even have the disease diagnosed. People in group D—true negatives—trade the relatively minor expense and inconvenience of being screened for the information that they are probably free of disease. If this reassurance is valuable, people in group D gain. However, screening may entail risks such as those in radiation. These risks could outweigh the value of reassurance. There may even be risks that are not known to the participants or to those doing the screening.

People in groups B and C suffer as a result of screening. False positives have to undergo a diagnostic evaluation that is the result of test error. This evaluation has financial costs, and it may be inconvenient and uncomfortable, lead to anxiety, or involve medical risks. False negatives are informed that they probably are healthy when, in fact, they are not. This false reassurance might lead someone to ignore disease symptoms when they do appear.

The relative proportions of gains and losses in a given screening program depend on the value of early treatment and the other conditions that determine the relative feasibility of the program. If the disease that is the target of the program is fairly prevalent and favorably affected by early treatment, then the number of people in group A_1 would be reasonably high. If, on the other hand, the prevalence of the disease and the specificity of the test are low, there would be excessive numbers in group B. Almost every disease for which screening is done is sufficiently rare that the actual numbers in group A_1, or even $A_1 + A_2$, would be less than those in groups B and C. That is, screening usually requires that many people accept fairly small adverse effects so that a few may achieve a great gain.

Sometimes one hears the opinion that it is wise to be screened fairly often in order "to be on the safe side." The above contrast of gains with adverse effects indicates that such a viewpoint is ill advised. A person who decides to be screened makes a bet, although all the information for a fully informed bet usually is not available. The stakes—extended life—are high, but the probability of winning is small. In order to have a chance of winning, one must face a somewhat larger chance of an adverse effect ranging from the minor to the serious, as well as accepting the cost of screening itself. If the chance of winning is virtually nil, the bet is a poor one.

The purpose of interpreting a decision to be screened as a bet is to emphasize the intimate relation between the epidemiologic characteristics of screening for a disease, and an individual decision to be screened. A rational decision must take into account all relevant information, not simply the desire to minimize one's probability of death from the disease. How often should a woman be screened for cervical cancer? Annual screening is often recommended. Because of the long natural history of preclinical cervical cancer, however, annual screening offers little advantage compared to screening every other year, or even every third year (see chapter 11). Thus, a woman would be unlikely in the extreme to have her life extended by the additional tests needed for annual, compared to somewhat less frequent, screening. Money spent for the additional tests would almost certainly be wasted. The additional tests would substantially increase the probability of at least one false positive result.

NOTES

[1]Although the criterion of positivity refers to the distribution of test results in diseased and well populations, the results of previous tests of the person being screened also could be taken into account. Before deciding whether a screening mammogram is positive or not, it might be compared to an earlier "baseline" examination (page 200). In principle, a test for growth retardation might compare present size to the individual's trend in growth (Cuckle and Wald, 1984). Little is known of the value of using previous information, but it could greatly increase the complexity or cost of screening.

[2]Assuming that the rate of progression of a disease is unrelated to its incidence rate, the sensitivity and specificity of risk indicators describe not only their ability to distinguish people who do (or do not) have preclinical disease but also their ability to distinguish people who will die of the disease from those who will not. Because of the difficulty in determining who truly has preclinical disease, this example focuses on the identification of people at high risk of death.

8 Formulation of Screening Policy: Response Curves and Determinants of Outcome

Much of this book is concerned with the types of observations and methods of analysis involved in estimating the effect that a program of early diagnosis and treatment has on the mortality or advanced morbidity rate from the disease of interest. The ultimate goal of such studies is a screening policy—a set of recommendations regarding the early detection and treatment of disease. The recommendations may be directed at an entire population or a special segment of it that is at high risk. A policy may be limited to a particular issue such as testing technique or frequency of application, or it may concern every operational aspect of detection and treatment.

A demonstration that a given program is effective is usually no more than the beginning of a screening policy. Nearly always there are questions of the benefit of screening more, or less, frequently; or in a broader, or narrower, age range; or in groups with different incidence rates; or in groups with different baseline levels of medical care; or with a different test, an improved test, or a combination of tests.

It is not possible to answer every such question of policy directly by observation of the effect of the corresponding screening on mortality or advanced morbidity. There are too many questions, and the cost in time, money, and personnel would be too high. If an answer is to be obtained reasonably fast from a study relating screening to mortality, the period of screening must be fairly short. Yet, the goal of the study may be to guide a policy of screening over most of adult life. How should the results of the study be used to formulate the policy? The HIP study showed that a program of four annual screenings by physical examination and mammography led to a particular reduction in mortality from breast cancer, but the study took 15 years, many millions of dollars, and involved 60,000 subjects, dozens of hospitals, and hundreds of professional personnel. What reduction in breast cancer mortality can be achieved with newer mammography techniques perhaps applied less frequently but over a longer period? What should be the role of physical examination or breast self-examination? Population screening for breast cancer is very expensive and may confer small but real risks to well people. It is crucial to design a screening policy that achieves a useful degree of control of breast cancer without placing an unreasonable economic or medical burden on the target population. The data needed to formulate all aspects of the policy with confidence are not in hand. To obtain the information directly would take many years and would be very expensive. Long before the answers were in, further improvements in screening and accumulating knowledge of breast cancer would inevitably render the results obsolete.

Therefore, attention has been given to indirect means of making the many decisions required to formulate screening policies. The term *model* is often used in this context. A model is a formal statement, often made in mathematical language, of the structure that is believed to explain a phenomenon or a set of observations. Some components of a model may be derived from algebraic relationships: Population age-specific mortality rates for a disease can be predicted if the age-specific incidence rates and subsequent rates of mortality among cases are known (Eddy, 1980; Morrison, 1979a). Typically, however, certain components have to be based on incomplete information, or, simply, intuition. For example, Schwartz (1978) assumed that the growth of breast cancer follows a particular equation, and he showed that a model incorporating this term made predictions that were consistent with observations on the stage of the disease at detection and mortality from the disease.

Most of the models of the diagnostic or therapeutic effects of screening that have been developed concern cancer. Investigators have made use of information on the distribution of lead time or the duration of preclinical disease. Eddy and Shwartz (1982) have reviewed mathematical models of cancer screening.

A good fit of a model to available data does not establish the general validity of the model but only that the data do not show the model to be *in*valid. The shape of the curve that relates amount of breast irradiation to the rate of breast cancer is of considerable interest and importance. It appears that a linear relation between the radiation dose in rads and the incidence rate of breast cancer is consistent with most observations that have been made, but more complex curves, such as a linear-quadratic model, also may fit the data (Boice et al, 1991). Some theoretical considerations suggest that the curve is concave upward at low doses. The nature of the curve bears on the risk of mammography. A small dose of radiation would lead to less breast cancer if the curve is concave upward rather than linear.

A model is most likely to give valid predictions when the situation being explored is similar to the one that generated the information used to construct the model. Suppose that a curve relating mortality rate to screening frequency is based on data from an experimental study that included groups with no screening, as well as screening every year and every three years. The model would probably yield reasonable predictions of the value of screening every two years. On the other hand, predictions of the value of screening every ten years, or screening with a different test (one that has uncertain sensitivity characteristics), would be questionable. In short, a prediction derived from a model is an hypothesis, not a scientific fact. To the extent that components of a model are of uncertain validity, its predictions should be regarded as tentative.

Two potentially useful methods of predicting the effects of screening involve response curves and intermediate determinants of outcome.

A response curve describes the relationship between the amount of an exposure and subsequent disease occurrence. A screening program can be characterized by exposure variables such as the frequency of examination, the age at which screening begins for an individual subject, and the length of the period over which a subject is screened. The frequency will often be the exposure variable of greatest interest. Given a sensitive test and an effective early treatment procedure, the curve relating reduction in mortality to the number of examinations evenly distributed in a broad age interval can be thought of, in general, as having a concave-downward shape (Figure 8–1). The initial portion of the curve would ascend relatively steeply, since an increase in the number of widely separated screening examinations would contribute a roughly proportional reduction in mortality. The steepness of this portion of the curve would depend on factors such as the incidence rate and duration of the preclinical phase, the curability of the disease, and the relationships of these factors to age. At high frequencies, the curve would be nearly flat, since the prevalence of cases detected in the later screens of a closely spaced series would be very low. Daily screening, for example, would lead to little reduction in mortality compared to monthly screening.

The portion of the curve encompassing the shift from steep to flat is most important is designing a screening program since the goal is to bring about a large reduction in mortality with as little screening and, therefore cost, as possible. An experimental screening program with two, or better, three properly chosen screening frequencies would give some indication of the characteristics of the curve. Selecting the screening frequencies to be evaluated will probably involve educated guesses based on knowledge of the natural history of the disease, and practical and economic considerations.

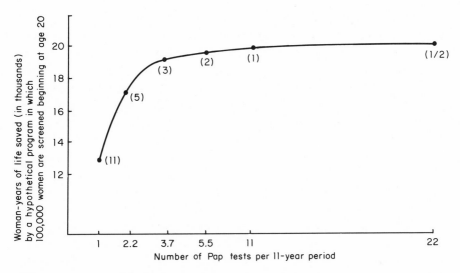

Figure 8–1. Example of a frequency-response relationship in screening.

Source: Adapted from American Cancer Society (1980).

The numbers in parentheses are the intervals (years) between examinations.

An upper limit of yearly screening would be a reasonable choice for many diseases. Yearly screening (1) is suited to health care schedules, (2) is probably the most frequent screening regarded as economically justified on a large scale, and (3) is probably frequent enough for a high proportion of preclinical cases of many chronic diseases to be detected. The lower frequencies will depend on the disease and the screening procedures under study. For example, the typical duration of carcinoma in situ of the cervix is thought to be many years long. Therefore, it might be reasonable to evaluate screening at intervals of five years or perhaps more. On the other hand, most cases of preclinical breast cancer may not be detectable for more than one to three years. Thus, screening at two-year intervals might be a good frequency to evaluate.

As estimate of the curve relating screening frequency to reduction in mortality would be a reasonable basis for translating data from experimental studies into policy decisions. Data from studies that enable such curves to be derived directly have not yet been reported, but Eddy (1980; American Cancer Society, 1980) used a simulation model to construct frequency-response curves related to screening for cancers of several sites. Given a schedule of screening with specified tests, expressions for the sensitivity characteristics of the tests are used together with age-specific incidence rates to predict the times of diagnosis of screen-detected and non-screen-detected cases. The effect of the program on mortality is predicted from the distribution of screening histories of diagnosed cases (eg, the numbers detected on the first screen, on subsequent screens, and in intervals between screens) and the corresponding case-fatality curves according to screening history.

As the purpose of this model is to predict the effect of a proposed program that has one or more features, such as frequency of screening, that have not been evaluated directly, the appropriate distribution of screening histories will not be known. Instead, the distribution that might be expected is derived from the results of programs, such as those with other frequencies, whose effects have been observed. It is likely that the sensitivity characteristics of screening or the value of early treatment would differ between a proposed new program and previous ones. Therefore, the number and timing of diagnoses of screen-detected cases, and case-fatality according to screening history, are likely to differ between the new program and those derived from earlier programs. The uncertainties in both distributions are potential sources of error in predictions based on the model, although such errors might be small.

Figure 8–1 is the frequency-response curve that was developed for cervical cancer. The curve suggests that screening at three-year intervals is substantially more effective than is screening at intervals of five years or greater. Even more frequent screening is of little additional value but would lead to greatly increased costs. Thus, screening at three-year intervals was proposed as a policy.

Decisions regarding the ages at which screening should begin and end may be guided by basic epidemiologic data on the disease and the frequency of other causes of death. Breast cancer, for example, is very uncommon before age 40. Thus, screening young women would be unrewarding unless a very early precursor of the illness were detectable and highly curable. Otherwise, few cases would be found, the predictive value of screening would be low, and its effect on mortality would be small. Although the incidence rate of breast cancer continues to increase with age in many countries, screening women above the age of, say, 75 or 80 may not be justified for another reason: The rates of death from other causes are so high that even a woman whose breast cancer is cured as a result of early detection is likely to die soon from an unrelated disease. The relation of breast cancer screening policy to age is considered in more detail in chapter 9.

In principle, many policy questions can be answered with knowledge of the functional relations between aspects of a screening schedule such as frequency, or ages of participants, and reduction in mortality. Our ability to make the necessary observations directly, however, is limited by the same practical factors that make evaluation of specific screening programs so difficult. The feasibility of evaluating the effects of screening can be increased by use of studies based on determinants of outcome—characteristics of the disease that can be assessed shortly after screening is done, typically at the time of diagnosis, and that predict subsequent changes in rates of death or serious morbidity. An experimental study, as described in chapter 4, involves both the diagnostic and subsequent therapeutic effects of a screening program. The use of determinants of outcome would allow evaluation to be based only on the diagnostic effects, provided that valid predictions of the therapeutic effects could be made. If so, various screening procedures and schedules—the core of screening policy—could be studied relatively quickly and cheaply. Studies based on determinants of outcome could be used to construct response curves that would be impractical to estimate directly.

The evolution of immunization methods for poliomeyelitis provides an excellent example of the use of a determinant of outcome. In early studies, it was shown that inoculation with inactivated virus leads to increased production of antibodies to the disease. A very large experimental study established the efficacy of inactivated-virus vaccine in preventing the disease (Francis et al, 1955). Later, a live attenuated-virus vaccine was developed that was, in several respects, more desirable than the earlier vaccine. It was not necessary to test the newer vaccine as extensively as the older one in order to document its efficacy. A study as large and rigorous as the Francis trial was not done again. Instead, attention was directed to finding a dose and a schedule of administration that lead to a sufficient antibody response, and to the evaluation of adverse effects of the vaccine (Bodian and Horstmann, 1965; Paul, 1963). The antibody titer produced by a given dose and schedule provided a satisfactory indication of subsequent resistance to polio. In the area of infectious disease control, antibody titer is a useful determinant of outcome because its relationship to risk of disease is readily assessed, and most or all of the preventive effect of immunization is known to be conveyed by the antibody titer. In other words, given the antibody titer, knowledge of immunization history adds little or no information about the pattern of risk with time.

Determinants of outcome reflect the mechanism by which the exposure acts. If screening is effective, it works by changing the point in the development of the disease at which it is treated. Therefore, the appropriate determinants reflect this change. Prediction of the efficacy of a new vaccine is based on its immunogenicity without explicit use of the vaccination histories of subjects. Similarly, predictions based on determinants of outcome do not make explicit use of the screening histories of diagnosed cases.

Stage at diagnosis is often considered as a determinant of cancer mortality. The difference in stage distribution between screened and unscreened groups can be thought of as being analagous to the difference in antibody titer between vaccinated and unvaccinated groups. The analogy would be valid if the efficacy of screening can be predicted accurately from a shift in stage. A shift to a more favorable stage distribution in a screened population has been taken as ipso facto evidence of ultimately reduced mortality. However, a shift in stage may reflect only lead time, and this type of analysis provides no information on the *size* of any reduction in mortality that is achieved.

A change in stage distribution also has been used to estimate the extent to which screening is associated with improved prognosis of diagnosed cases. Foster et al (1978) investigated self-examination for breast cancer. They found substantial differences in the distribution of stage at diagnosis according to whether the cases reported performing breast self-examination monthly, less than monthly, or never. Five stages based on the size of the tumor and the degree of spread were used with these distributions; Foster et al then predicted five-year survival probabilities for each group by applying the respective stage distribution as a set of weights to stage-specific survival figures obtained from standard sources (Table 8–1). Thus, a five-year survival of 76% was predicted for cases who performed monthly self-examination, 69% survival for those who did self-examination less often than monthly, and 59% for those who never used the procedure.

Table 8–1. Percentage Distribution of Stage at Diagnosis of Breast Cancer, and Predicted Five-Year Survival, According to Frequency of Breast Self-examination

Frequency of self-examination	Percent in stage						Predicted five-year survival (%)
	0	I	II	III	IV	All stages	
Monthly (60)[a]	5.0	50.0	40.0	5.0	0.0	100.0	76[b]
Less than monthly (68)	2.9	32.4	50.0	13.2	1.5	100.0	69
Never (117)	0.9	17.9	43.6	33.3	4.3	100.0	59
Expected five-year survival (%)	100	85	66	41	10	—	—

Source: Foster RS Jr, Lang SP, Costanza MC, Worden JK, Haines CR, Yates JW: Breast self-examination practices and breast-cancer stage. *N Engl J Med* 1978:229:265–270. Reprinted by permission of the New England Journal of Medicine.

[a]Numbers of patients are given in parentheses.

[b]Value was derived as follows: 5.0 (100) + 50.0 (85) + 40.0 (66) + 5.0 (41) + 0.0 (10) = 76.

This approach is attractive because of its simplicity, but it is not possible to distinguish the effects of lead time or pseudodisease on survival from a true reduction in mortality. Early detection, even without any accompanying extension of life, would lead to an improvement in the predicted case survival. This possibility is illustrated by the results from the Mayo Clinic study of lung cancer given in chapter 4. Early detection favorably altered the stage distribution. Had the data on stage been used to predict survival, this also would have been improved in the screened group since survival is better for localized compared to nonlocalized lung cancer, and the observed survival was higher for cases in the screened group. Nonetheless, comparison of the screened and unscreened populations showed that mortality from lung cancer was virtually unchanged by intensive screening. In short, determinants of mortality or advanced morbidity may not, by themselves, be valid outcome variables. Prorok et al (1981) referred to stage as a "pseudovariable."

Determinants of outcome *can* be used in appropriate circumstances to make valid *predictions* of the effect of screening (Morrison, 1991b). The date of death of each case—basic data for estimation of the mortality rate by time—is determined by the date of diagnosis of the case and its period of survival. Suppose that the time at which death from the disease in that case will occur, if at all, is indicated with little or no error by the extent of the disease at the time of diagnosis and initial treatment. The extent of a cancer might be assessed by its size, the number of positive lymph nodes, and the locations and sizes of distant metastases. The lead time gained by each screen-detected case would correspond nearly perfectly to the change in extent, compared to what it would have been without screening. The disease-specific mortality by time in a population could be predicted by linking the time of diagnosis of each case to its expected time of death, given the extent. The effect of screening on mortality could be estimated accurately by comparing predicted mortality between screened and unscreened groups, based on the times of diagnosis of cases and their expected times of death, given prognostic characteristics.

Prognostic characteristics that indicate precisely the time of death for individual cases are not known; there is substantial uncertainty in the prognosis of an individual with a given set of prognostic variables. Nonetheless, known prognostic factors for many diseases do have strong effects on the distribution of time of death. For example, the five-year case fatality in breast cancer is 12% for patients with no involved lymph nodes, compared to 43% for patients with four or more involved nodes (Ries L; unpublished data from the Surveillance, Epidemiology and End Results program). Since case-fatality data according to stage are widely available for cancer, mortality can be predicted by applying stage-specific case-fatality curves to the times of diagnosis of cases in the screened and unscreened groups. Much of the discussion that follows concerns screening for cancer, but the ideas are applicable to any disease for which there are prognostic factors that change with time during the development of the disease.

The relation between the incidence of and mortality from a disease in a population that is eligible to be screened but is not being screened is given in chapter 2. M_T is the population cumulative mortality for year T, the number of deaths from the disease in the interval divided by the total number of persons alive at the start of the interval. For simplicity, this presentation focuses on the numerators, designated as D_T. These are all that are necessary for estimation of the effect of screening in an experiment with groups of equal size. If the groups are not equal, the D_T's may be adjusted to compensate for the difference in the sizes of the groups.

Let

$C_{a.}$ = number of persons diagnosed during year a after the start of observation

$f_{j.}$ = conditional cumulative case fatality from the disease during year j after diagnosis

$f_{T-a+1.}$ = conditional cumulative case fatality from the disease during year T after the start of observation, among cases diagnosed during year a after the start of observation

D_T = number of cases that die during year T after the start of observation

Then

$$D_T = \sum_{a=1}^{T} f_{T-a+1.} \left[\prod_{j=0}^{T-a} (1 - f_j) \right] C_a \qquad (8-1)$$

Next, imagine a set of prognostic categories indexed by the subscript k. The term *stage* is used to describe a set of such prognostic factors. If the stage is based on tumor size (small or large) and spread to regional lymph nodes (no or yes), k might take the values 1 (small, no), 2 (small, yes), 3 (large, no), and 4 (large, yes).

If $C_{a,k}$ = the number of cases diagnosed during year a that have a given value of k, then D_T can be written as a sum over the k stages.

$$D_T = \sum_{k} \left\{ \sum_{a=1}^{T} f_{T-a+1,k} \left[\prod_{j=0}^{T-a} (1 - f_{j,k}) \right] C_{a,k} \right\} \qquad (8-2)$$

Expression (8-2) is the basic prediction equation. In it, the number of deaths from the disease is shown to depend on the times of diagnosis and stages of the cases (given by the $C_{a,k}$), and stage-specific case fatalities (the

$f_{j,k}$). A change in D_T that is the result of early detection and treatment could be predicted from the $C_{a,k}$ in a screened group and in a comparable unscreened group provided that the appropriate $f_{j,k}$ are known from another source. Typically, the $f_{j,k}$ would be assumed to be constant with calendar time.

In predictions based on determinants of mortality, the lead times correspond to the changes in the prognostic factors on which the predictions depend. A relatively low stage, and the accompanying low case fatality, might reflect lead time (early diagnosis) but not a greater effect of treatment than would be conferred on the same cases if they had been diagnosed later. This would be true if the outcome of the disease is determined very early in its course, before any cases are diagnosed. If so, screening will not be beneficial over the range of stages that would be used to predict the effect of screening. If there is a beneficial effect of screening and it is to be predicted accurately by stage at diagnosis, the change in stage that is created by screening must account entirely for the lead time as well as for the entire beneficial effect of early treatment on case fatality. Furthermore, the relation between stage and case fatality must be identical in screened and unscreened persons irrespective of whether the disease is screen-detected (Morrison, 1985, page 165; Prentice, 1989).

Predictions of the effect of screening based on determinants of mortality can be made by use of either experimental or nonexperimental methods. In an experiment, the time at which each subject either does, or does not, become eligible for screening is known by design (randomization or invitation), and diagnoses are timed with respect to this point. In a nonexperimental study such a point must be defined by the investigator (see chapter 5). For example, it may be the age at which subjects first become eligible for screening, with the screened group being those who are actually screened at that age. Once this point is defined, application with the follow-up design is straightforward and corresponds to an experiment. In the case-control method, newly diagnosed cases are identified, timed with respect to screening, and classified as to the prognostic factors. The times of death are predicted, and the predicted deaths become the cases for analysis.

The use of determinants of outcome is illustrated with data from the HIP study (Morrison, 1991b). The goals of the analysis were to predict the reduction in deaths from breast cancer within ten years of entry, based on the characteristics of cases diagnosed within the first five years, and to compare the predicted reduction with the observed reduction. The analysis was only carried up to ten years from the start of observation because the basic results of the HIP study did not change much with further follow-up, and because case-fatality data, a crucial component of the method of prediction, usually are not available for periods of more than ten years after diagnosis. For the purpose of illustrating and evaluating the method, case-fatality data were derived from the experience of cases in the HIP control group. Case-fatality curves were expressed as one-year conditional cumulative probabilities of death from all causes for each of the first ten years after diagnosis. Breast cancer deaths were defined as deaths from all causes among breast cancer cases.

In typical predictions made by use of intermediate determinants of outcome, stage-specific case fatality data (the $f_{j,k}$) from outside the study would be used, since the point of the method is to predict the reduction in mortality without long-term observation of subjects in the study. As a result of self-selection, subjects in a study might have case fatalities that differ from those used to predict subsequent mortality. Such differences, however, are not likely to have much influence on the predicted effects of screening.

The cumulative numbers of observed deaths from breast cancer in the control group during the first ten years after entry are compared to the numbers predicted, without consideration of prognostic variables, in Table 8–2. The predicted values are derived from the numbers of cases according to time of diagnosis (C_a) and the case fatalities (f_j) of all cases combined. The differences between the observed and predicted numbers of deaths are small. The probable source of these differences is random variability in case fatality with time. Expressions (8–1) and (8–2) assume that the f_j and $f_{j,k}$ are constant with time for the duration of the study.

Table 8–2. Observed and Predicted Breast Cancer Deaths[a] in Controls, by Year after Entry

Year after entry	Cumulative deaths from breast cancer	
	Observed	Predicted
1	3	3.1
2	9	12.4
3	21	26.5
4	42	44.0
5	68	65.4
6	94	86.8
7	113	104.5
8	123	118.7
9	136	129.7
10	144	138.7

Source: Morrison (1991b).

[a]All deaths among breast cancer cases diagnosed within five years of entry in the HIP study.

Predicted reductions in deaths were then derived by calculating cumulative numbers of deaths for both the study group, including both compliers and noncompliers, and the control group. Each estimate made use of the stage-specific case fatalities as derived from the control group (the $f_{j,k}$) and the times of diagnosis (the $f_{a,k}$) for the screened group or the control group. If the predicted and observed reductions in the study group are the same, this implies that a beneficial effect of screening, assuming that one exists, is completely explained by the change created by screening in times of diagnosis and prognostic characteristics of cases.

Predictions were made with different means of categorizing stage at diagnosis (Table 8–3). The first set of predictions incorporated only a crude measure of stage: axillary lymph nodes negative, positive, or unknown. From the third year onward, the predicted reduction in breast cancer deaths was consistently and substantially less than that observed (Table 8–2). After ten years, the predicted reduction was 8.4 deaths compared to an observed reduction of 31 deaths. The second set of predictions made use of stage as assessed by the HIP from the hospital record. Six categories were used: local, regional, local extension, and metastatic (based on pathologic evidence), clinical stages local or regional (without evidence of local extension or metastasis), and unknown. The predicted reductions were similar to the previous ones and again substantially less than the

Table 8–3. Predicted Cumulative Control-study Difference in Deaths from Breast Cancer[a] by Year after Entry, Using Lymph Node Status and Stage as Early Outcomes

Year after entry	Difference in deaths as predicted by use of	
	Lymph node status	Stage
1	−1.6	−2.3
2	−1.0	−3.2
3	0.1	−1.7
4	0.4	−1.9
5	2.6	0.7
6	5.3	3.9
7	7.1	6.4
8	8.0	7.9
9	8.3	8.6
10	8.4	8.8

Source: Morrison (1991b).

[a]All deaths among breast cancer cases diagnosed within five years of entry in the HIP study.

observed reductions. An additional analysis was done with a measure of the extent of cancer that made use of information on the size of the tumor and the number of positive lymph nodes. The predictions obtained, however, were similar to those described above.

Table 8–4 compares seven-year case fatality between cases in the study and control groups. Lymph node status and stage are categorized as they were for the predictions given in Table 8–3. The seven-year case fatality is presented because the average period of follow-up used in the ten-year prediction was between seven and eight years. For both lymph node status and stage, the category-specific case fatality was higher in the control group than it was in the study group. The difference between control and study groups is especially large for regional-stage cases, and there is a corresponding difference among cases with positive lymph node status.

Table 8–4 also presents the proportions of cases in the study and control groups according to the pathologic category in which they were diagnosed.

Table 8–4. Seven-year Case Fatality[a] and Distribution of Cases[b] for Study and Control Groups According to Lymph Node Status and According to Stage

Early outcome	Group	
	Study	Control
Lymph node status		
negative	.189 (.559)	.234 (.450)
positive	.513 (.345)	.597 (.409)
unknown	.634 (.095)	.761 (.141)
Total (crude)	.343	.457
Total (adjusted)[c]	.343	.409
Stage		
local	.186 (.599)	.222 (.446)
regional	.453 (.293)	.566 (.342)
local extension	.893 (.059)	.804 (.104)
metastatic	1.000 (.039)	1.000 (.036)
clinically local or regional	.188 (.039)	.368 (.043)
unknown	.833 (.010)	1.000 (.029)
Total (crude)	.344	.457
Total (adjusted)[c]	.344	.401

Source: Morrison (1991b).

[a]All deaths among breast cancer cases diagnosed within five years of entry in the HIP study.

[b]Given in parentheses.

[c]Adjusted by use of weights from study group.

As expected, more cases in the study group were lymph node negative, and fewer were lymph node positive, compared to the control group. Similarly, there was a higher proportion of local stage cases, and lower proportions of regional and local extension cases in the study group compared to the control group. The proportion of metastatic cases was low in each group.

Finally, Table 8–4 compares the overall seven-year case fatality between cases in the study and control groups. The comparisons are made with and without adjustment for the proportion of cases according to lymph node status or stage. For each method of classification, adjustment reduced the control-study difference in case fatality, compared to the crude difference. Neither adjustment, however, entirely accounted for the difference in case fatality between the two groups. The effect of adjustment is similar for lymph node status and stage. Categorization of cases according to the actual number of involved lymph nodes (0,1,2,3, or 4+) and corresponding adjustment also did not explain the crude control-study difference in case fatality.

Table 8–5 gives the cumulative numbers of breast cancer deaths according to the stage at diagnosis of the cases. The numbers of deaths in cases that originally were local stage were identical in the two groups, although, as noted above, there were more local stage cases in the study group than were in the control group. All the originally metastatic cases in each group died. There were five more deaths in the study group than in the control

Table 8–5. Observed Cumulative Number of Deaths from Breast Cancer[a] 10 Years after Entry and Number of Cases[b] According to Stage at Diagnosis and Assigned Group

	Group			
Stage	Study		Control	
local	36	(170)	36	(133)
regional	43	(89)	65	(104)
local extension	16	(18)	27	(34)
metastatic	12	(12)	7	(7)
clinically local or regional	3	(12)	3	(14)
unknown	3	(3)	6	(6)
Total	113	(304)	144	(298)

Source: (Morrison, 1991b).

[a]All deaths among breast cancer cases diagnosed within five years of entry in the HIP study

[b]The numbers diagnosed within five years of entry are given in parentheses.

group from this source. The major source of the control-study reduction in deaths was cases that had been diagnosed as regional stage. As shown in Table 8–4, there was a large control study difference in case fatality in this category.

There are several reasons why predictions of the effect of screening that are based on determinants of mortality may not be entirely accurate. Most types of error are likely to create underestimation of the effect.

First, the change in distribution of a prognostic variable brought about by screening might not be highly correlated with lead time or with the change in case fatality owing to early treatment. Death from most types of cancer is the result of metastasis, not the primary tumor. Case fatality depends very strongly on whether the primary cancer is treated before metastasis occurs. The vast majority of patients with known distant metastases die within a few months or years.

Most deaths among cancer patients, however, are not derived from those who have known distant metastases at the time of diagnosis. Presumably the deaths are the results of metastases that were present but too small to be detected at the time of diagnosis and treatment. An ideal determinant of mortality would reflect the presence and treatability of such metastases. Prognostic variables, such as size of primary tumor and number of positive lymph nodes, function as indicators of the likelihood that an undetected metastasis has occurred. Such variables are not perfectly correlated with either the existence of metastases or their treatability. A case with involved lymph nodes may or may not have a distant but undetected metastasis. A beneficial effect of screening might be derived, in part, from a reduction in the frequency of undetected metastases among cases with a given degree of involvement of the lymph nodes. If so, the difference in degree of lymph node involvement between cases in screened and unscreened groups will not explain the entire beneficial effect of screening, and case fatality given the degree of lymph node involvement will differ between cases in the two groups. It is possible that no amount of refinement of technique for assessing the involvement of lymph nodes can eliminate this error.

Second, there may be variation of the prognostic factors within the measurement categories that are used. An extreme, although common, example is the categorization of anywhere from one to 50 or more positive lymph nodes as regional stage. Even when the number of positive nodes is given exactly, the volume of tumor for a given number of positive nodes may vary and the volume may itself be an important prognostic factor. A screen-detected case, which might have fewer involved nodes or a lower volume of tumor as a result of lead time, might be assigned to the same stage as it would have been without early detection. If cases in the screened group have a more favorable within-category distribution of prognostic factors than cases in the unscreened group, the stage-specific case fatality of cases in the screened group will be lower than that of cases in the control group, and the reduction in mortality from screening will be underpredicted.

Third, there may be measurement error in the assessment of the prognostic factor, the error being the same for cases in the screened and unscreened groups. The size of the primary tumor might not be correctly measured, or the stated number of metastases in regional lymph nodes might be incorrect. As a result of such errors, the difference in distribution of stage between screened and unscreened groups will not completely account for the lead time of screening and any consequent benefit. Furthermore, the prognostic factor will explain less of the variability in case fatality than it would if measured without error. Thus, the predicted change in mortality as a result of screening would tend to be less than the actual change.

Fourth, the accuracy of prediction would be affected if the quality of measurement of prognostic variables differs between screened and unscreened groups. Depending on the nature of the errors, the effect of screening may be underpredicted or overpredicted. Differences in data quality are unlikely to occur in an experiment or in a nonexperimental study if the data on screened and unscreened subjects are derived from the same sources, eg, the records of a prepaid medical plan. In even the best designed study, however, the frequency of missing data on stage may differ between groups. For example, low-stage cases, who are more likely to have been screened, might be less likely than higher-stage cases to have lymph nodes removed for examination. A possible solution to this problem is to consider *unknown* as a separate stage. Even so, the observed treatment effect may differ between screened and unscreened patients of unknown stage.

The effect of treatment at a given stage might differ for screen-detected v nonscreen-detected cases, because screening preferentially identifies cases that are more (or less) susceptible to treatment than are unscreened cases at the same stage. Depending on the interrelation of stage, mode of detection, and effect of treatment, there may be either over or underprediction of the change in mortality from screening.

There might be an improvement in treatment during the time that a study of screening is in progress. A prediction of the effect of screening based on case-fatality data from an earlier period obviously could not take account of the recent improvement. Depending on the relation of the improvement to the extent of the disease, the improvement might either increase or decrease the value of screening.

Screening may lead to the detection of pseudodisease (page 24). Unless the treatment of such cases is in some way harmful, the detection of pseudodisease has no effect on the *observed* difference in mortality between screened and unscreened groups. By definition, the case fatality of pseudodisease is zero. If the prognostic features of pseudodisease, such as in situ cancer, are known, then pseudodisease will not affect the accuracy of prediction. It is possible, however, that pseudodisease cannot be distinguished from some types of more serious disease that lead to symptomatic illness. If so, the corresponding case fatality as estimated from routinely available data will be too high. The result will be an underestimation of the reduction in mortality brought about by early treatment.

Prognostic selection refers to the possible tendency of screening to identify cases that have an unusual prognosis irrespective of the lead time or the (average) beneficial effect of early treatment. A frequently described example of prognostic selection bias is length bias (pages 142 to 147). As a result of length bias, case fatality measured from diagnosis might differ between screen-detected and nonscreen-detected cases in a screened population, but length bias does not affect a comparison of case fatality between *all* cases in screened *v* unscreened populations. Therefore, comparisons of mortality between screened and unscreened populations will not be affected by length bias.

In the analysis of the HIP data, screening was predicted to reduce mortality from breast cancer, but the predicted benefit was substantially less than the benefit that was observed. Had the predictions been accurate, the control-study difference in the distribution of prognostic factors would have been greater than was observed, and the prognostic-factor specific case fatalities would have been equal for cases in the two groups. In fact, the case fatalities differed between the study and control groups within categories of the prognostic variables that were used. Thus, changes in the prognostic variables as measured do not entirely account for the effect of screening in reducing mortality. The data do suggest, however, that the beneficial effect of screening was the result of the early treatment of cases that otherwise would have been relatively advanced at diagnosis. Few noninvasive cases were detected in either group (Shapiro et al, 1988), so most of the benefit could not have been derived from the detection of noninvasive disease.

The results suggest that the predictions were affected by one or more of the types of errors described. Neither the accuracy of prediction nor the control-study differences in case fatality was influenced much by increasing the number of categories or changing the type of prognostic variable used in the analysis. This finding indicates that (1) the different classification systems (ie, lymph node status *v* stage) provide similar information on the change in the true extent of disease as related to early treatment, and (2) control-study differences in the distributions of determinants of mortality within categories of lymph node status or stage were not an important source of error. With the present material it is not possible to distinguish the sizes of errors related to inaccurate measurement of prognostic factors v imperfect correlation of the factors with the presence and treatability of metastases.

Some more recent data are consistent with the results derived from the HIP. The Breast Cancer Detection Demonstration Project (BCDDP) was a nationwide program in which the screening was done between 1973 and 1981. Breast cancer mortality among participants in this program was somewhat lower than expected, which is consistent with a beneficial effect of the program (Morrison et al, 1988). For all breast cancers (screen-detected or not) that were diagnosed within five years of entry, the five-year case fatality was 6.5% for invasive cases without lymph node involvements, 13.1% for cases with one to three nodes involved, and 28.3% for cases with four or more nodes involved. "Unscreened" comparison data on case fatality were derived from the Surveillance, Epidemiology, and End Results (SEER) program for cases diagnosed in the years 1977 to 1982 (Reis L; unpublished data). The respective category-specific case fatalities were 11.6%, 21.2%, and 43.0%. Thus, as with the HIP, screened-unscreened differences in case fatality are seen within categories of a prognostic factor. If the SEER case-fatality data were to be used in conjunction with the dates of diagnosis and distribution of involved nodes in the BCDDP, the effect of screening on mortality would again be underpredicted.

The size of a reduction in mortality, not merely its existence, is crucial information in the evaluation of screening. For example, the balance of the cancer-control value v the adverse effects and costs of screening may differ greatly for a reduction of eight or nine deaths v 31 deaths out of a total of 144. Therefore, it is important to learn whether the error of prediction can be substantially reduced by more careful measurement of prognostic variables, or, perhaps, the use of different or additional variables. If so, predictions based on intermediate determinants of mortality could make a useful contribution to the evaluation of screening.

9 Cancer of the Breast

The HIP project stimulated many additional studies of the early detection and treatment of breast cancer. As a result, screening for breast cancer has been investigated more thoroughly than any other type of screening to control a progressive chronic disease. The most important of these studies are experiments to evaluate screening that includes mammography, with or without professional physical examination of the breast. These studies are reviewed and interpreted first. Next, nonexperimental studies of screening by mammography with or without physical examination are reviewed and summarized. Then, findings on self-examination of the breasts are presented and discussed. Finally, a series of overall conclusions and implications of the findings for screening policy are given.

This chapter is derived from Morrison (1989). The studies considered are limited to those that relate screening to breast cancer mortality or, in one instance, advanced invasive breast cancer.

EXPERIMENTAL STUDIES

Methods and results

These studies are summarized in Table 9–1.

THE HIP (HEALTH INSURANCE PLAN) STUDY (Shapiro et al, 1988): This study is described in detail in chapter 4. It began in 1963. Women who were 40 to 64 years old were enrolled. Subjects were randomized individually. The study group (n = 30,131) was eligible for a program of four screening examinations that included mammography and breast palpation. The

Table 9-1. Summary of Experimental Studies of the Effect of Screening on Breast Cancer Mortality

Study	Type of screening and frequency	Age at entry (years)	Number of subjects	Percent compliance at first screen	Length of follow-up (years)	Percent reduction in breast cancer mortality
HIP Shapiro et al (1988)	Two-view mammography and breast palpation annually	40–64	30,131 study 30,565 control	65	7	33
Two County (Sweden) Tabar et al (1985, 1989)	Single-view mammography[a]	40–74	77,080 study 55,985 control	89	7.9	30
UK[b] UK Trial Group (1981, 1988)	Single-view or two-view mammography every two years; breast palpation annually	45–64	45,841 study 127,117 control	66	6.6	20
Malmo Andersson et al (1988)	Single-view or two-view mammography every 18–24 months	45–69	21,088 study 21,195 control	74	8.8	4
Edinburgh Roberts et al (1990)	Single-view or two-view mammography every two years; breast palpation every two years	45–64	23,226 study 21,904 control	61	7	17
Stockholm Frisell et al (1991)	Single-view mammography about every 28 months	40–64	40,318 study 19,943 control	80	7.4	29

[a]The intervals between examinations were about 24 months for women aged 40–49 and 33 months for women aged 50 and above.
[b]This was an intervention study without random assignment.

examinations were planned to be done annually. The control group (n = 30,565) was eligible for regular check-ups that were available, if desired, through the HIP. Sixty-five per cent of the screened group had at least the first examination; 39% had all four. The proportion of the control group that had physical examinations has not been reported. A difference in breast cancer mortality in favor of screening was first clearly apparent after four years. After seven years, the cumulative mortality from breast cancer was reduced 33% in the study group compared to the control group, based on cases diagnosed within five years of entry (Relative Risk = 0.67). Early in the study, there was little effect of screening among women 40 to 49 years of age at entry. After five years, the RR was 0.95 for these women, compared to an RR of 0.47 for women 50 to 64. An effect of screening in younger women appeared after about ten years. After 14 years, the RR was 0.75 for women 40 to 49 years of age at entry and the RR was 0.78 for women 50 to 64.

THE TWO COUNTY (SWEDEN) STUDY (Tabar et al, 1985, 1989): The study began in 1977. The women enrolled were 40 to 74 years old. Subjects were randomized by area of residence within each county. The study group (n = 77,080) was eligible for single-view mammography. The first two examinations were done on an average of 24 months apart for women who were 40 to 49 years old, and an average of 33 months apart for women who were 50 years of age or older. Later examinations were done at average intervals of 22 months for women under 50 and 24 months for older women (Fagerberg and Tabar, 1988). There were 55,985 women in the control group. Compliance at the first screen was 89% (93% in women 40 to 49 years old; 79% in women 70 to 74 years old); at the second screen, 83% of all members of the study group still living in the study area participated (89% of women 40 to 49 years old; 67% of women 70 to 74 years old). After an average of six years of follow-up, 13% of the control group had had mammography, mostly near the end of the period. A difference in breast cancer mortality in favor of screening was first clearly apparent after five years. With an average of 7.9 years of follow-up, the cumulative mortality from breast cancer was 30% lower in the study group than it was in the control group (RR = 0.70; 0.55–0.87, 95% confidence interval). The effect of screening was almost entirely concentrated among older women. The RR was 0.92 (0.52–1.60) for women 40 to 49 years of age at entry, the RR was 0.60 (0.40–0.90) for women 50 to 59, the RR was 0.65 (0.44–0.95) for women 60 to 69, and the RR was 0.77 (0.47–1.27) for women 70 to 74 years of age at entry.

THE UK TRIAL (UK Trial of Early Detection of Cancer Group, 1988): This study began in 1979. The women enrolled were 45 to 64 years old. Subjects were not randomized; the screening for which they were eligible depended on their area of residence. Women in the two screening districts (n = 45,841) were offered annual physical examination and biennial mammography for seven years. Two-view mammography was used in one of the areas; single-view mammography was used in the other one (UK Trial of Early Detection of Cancer Group, 1981). There were two breast self-examination (BSE) districts. Women in these districts (n = 63,636) were offered class instruction in breast self-examination at the start of the study, and a self-referral clinic was provided. There were four control districts. The women living there (n = 127,117) were eligible for regularly available medical care. In the screening districts, compliance at the first screen was at least 66%, and at least 59% at the fifth examination. (The estimates are minimums because of inaccuracies in population registers.) At least 44% of the BSE group had the class instruction that was offered. The extent to which women in the control districts were screened is not known. A difference in breast cancer mortality in favor of screening was first clearly apparent after six years of observation. After an average of 6.6 years, the cumulative mortality from breast cancer was reduced 20% in the screening districts (RR = 0.80; 0.64–1.01) and increased four percent in the BSE districts (RR = 1.04; 0.86–1.26). These values were adjusted for the pretrial breast cancer mortality rates in the respective areas. Data on mortality were not given by age.

THE MALMO TRIAL (Andersson et al, 1988): The study began in 1976. The women enrolled were 45 to 69 years old. Subjects were randomized individually. The study group (n = 21,088) was eligible for mammography (two-view in the first two examinations; subsequently one-view for mammographically fatty breasts, or two-view for dense breasts). Examinations were done every 18 to 24 months; five examinations were completed. There were 21,195 women in the control group. In the study group, compliance at the first screen was 74% (79% in women 45 to 49 years old; 64% in women 75 to 79 years old); compliance was 70% at later screens. In the control group, an estimated 24% had mammography during the study (35% of women 45 to 49 years of age at entry; 13% of women 65 to 69). For the first six years, the annual numbers of breast cancer deaths were higher in the study than in the control group. Later annual differences were in the opposite direction. At the end of the period of follow-up (an average of 8.8 years) the RR was 0.96 (0.68–1.35). For women 55 years and older at entry, the RR was 0.79 (0.51–1.24). For women less than 55 at entry, the RR was 1.29 (0.74–2.25).

THE EDINBURGH TRIAL (Roberts et al, 1990): The study began in 1979. The women enrolled were 45 to 64 years old. The subjects were randomized according to the general practices in which they were enrolled. The study group (n = 23,226) was eligible for annual screening. The first examination included two-view mammography and breast palpation. Palpation alone was done at the second, fourth, and sixth examinations. Single-view mammography and palpation was done at the third, fifth, and seventh examinations. The control group included 21,904 women. In the study group, compliance at the first screen was 61.3% (63.8% in women 45 to 49 years of age; 56.5% in women 60 to 64). Compliance at the third screen was 51.3% (55.9% in women 45 to 49; 47.6% in women 60 to 64). The extent of screening in the control group was not reported. From the second through sixth years of observation, breast cancer mortality was slightly lower among study than control women. The difference increased somewhat in the seventh year. After seven years, the RR was 0.83 (0.57–1.18), with adjustment for age. Among women 50 years of age and older at entry, the RR was 0.80 (0.54–1.17)

THE STOCKHOLM TRIAL (Frisell et al, 1991): The study began in 1981. The women enrolled were 40 to 64 years old. The subjects were randomized individually. The study group (n = 40,318) was eligible for single-view mammography. Two examinations were done an at average of about 28 months apart. There were 19,943 women in the control group. Compliance was approximately 80% at each examination, and compliance was nearly constant with age. Twenty-five percent of women in the study group had had a mammogram during the three-year period before the study. The women in the control group were invited to be screened once at an average time of about four and one-half years after entry; compliance at this examination was 77%. A modest difference in breast cancer mortality in favor of screening was apparent after two years of observation. The difference became somewhat larger after six years. After an average of 7.4 years of observation, the cumulative mortality from breast cancer was reduced an average of 29% in the study group compared to the control group (RR = 0.71; 0.4–1.2). For women 50 to 64 years of age at entry, the RR was 0.57 (0.3–1.1). For women 40 to 49 years of age at entry, the RR was 1.09 (0.4–3.0).

Interpretation

These results are reasonably compatible in showing a beneficial effect of screening on breast cancer mortality in women at least 45, 50, or 55 years of age at entry. Nonetheless, there are several aspects of these studies and their results that bear on the formulation of screening policy for breast cancer.

SCREENING METHODS: The HIP study used two tests—mammography and (professional) physical examination—and there is no direct way to separate their effects on breast cancer mortality in that study. There was, however, indirect evidence that physical examination made a contribution to the effect of screening (Table 3–2). In recent studies, mammography has received more attention than physical examination. Improvements in mammographic technology might reduce the relative value of physical examination in a program of combined screening, but there is no reason to expect a program of mammographic screening alone to have the same effect as a combined program unless mammography detects every case that physical examination would find.

SCREENING SCHEDULE (frequency and duration): In the HIP study, women were screened annually for a maximum of four examinations (ie, a three-year period of screening). There has been no intervention study of screening done more frequently than yearly. In the studies that followed the HIP, screening was done at intervals ranging from one year to nearly three years. Other things being equal, when screening is done less frequently, the reduction in mortality is smaller. The shape of the curve that relates frequency to mortality is not known, but it probably is not linear (see chapter 8). Changes of frequency within certain limits might result in only slight differences in the value of screening. For example, screening every year might be only slightly better than screening every 18 months or even every two years.

The duration of the screening program was more than three years in recent studies. In some studies, the screening has been continued indefinitely. The effects on mortality of such differences in the duration of screening may be difficult to measure with less than, say, ten years of observation.

STUDY SIZE: Although large populations have been studied, the *effective* sample sizes are small because only a small fraction of those screened have detectable asymptomatic breast cancer. In the HIP study, for example, there were 132 breast cancers detected among 20,000 women who were screened, many of them repeatedly. The entire difference in breast cancer mortality between the study and control groups is derived from the early treatment of those 132 cases. The precision of differences in breast cancer mortality, as observed in the studies described, is relatively poor, as shown by the wide confidence intervals. Thus, observed effects of screening are likely to vary from study to study even if the underlying true effect is constant. Estimates of the effects of screening in narrow age intervals are subject to substantially more random error than are the overall results. It is not clear that any of the studies reported to date are large enough to provide a precise estimate of a *difference* in the effect of screening younger *v* older women.

SCREENING TECHNOLOGY: Mammographic technique has improved recently (Kopans et al, 1984). There is likely to have been a corresponding decrease in the size of tumors that can be detected (Alexander et al, 1990; Silverstein et al, 1989). It might be assumed that this change would result in a reduction in breast cancer mortality. The detection and early treatment of tumors when they are very small, however, might not make much difference compared to detecting them when they are somewhat larger.

SCREENING QUALITY: Assuming a constant level of technology, it is most unlikely that screening by either mammography or physical examination has been done with similar levels of skill in every study. The extent of central coordination and quality control might also affect the quality of screening.

"BACKGROUND" SCREENING: Screening takes place in a context of a particular level of medical care and "health-awareness." The effect of a given program depends on the circumstances in which it is implemented. The HIP program would have had a much smaller effect than it did if it had been evaluated in a setting in which intensive screening for breast cancer was already a standard part of medical care. In recent years, it is likely that breast cancer has been diagnosed and treated increasingly early as a result of generally increasing participation in medical care, decreasing reluctance of women to seek attention for breast symptoms, and the increasing use of mammography and breast examination by physicians. These changes imply that the measurable effect of a new program based on current methods of screening is likely to diminish as time passes and background screening becomes more prevalent.

COMPLIANCE OF STUDY SUBJECTS: Compliance of the screened group was highest in the Two County study, and next highest in the Stockholm trial. Compliance was similar for the HIP and UK and Edinburgh studies. Compliance tended to be higher in relatively young women. The compliance (ie, lack of screening) in the control group depends on the level of background screening. As might be expected, the compliance of controls has decreased with time. In the Malmo study, nearly a quarter of the controls had mammography during the study. In the Stockholm trial, a quarter of the women invited to be screened had been screened recently, and the controls were offered screening late in the trial. Thus, the differences in the amount of screening between the study and control groups in these studies were relatively small.

LENGTH OF OBSERVATION: In the studies with overall positive results, the reported reductions in breast cancer mortality varied from 17% to 33%. The effect of screening is not constant with time after the start of a program. The effect depends on the natural history of the disease and the way in which early treatment changes it. In the studies described, at least four or five years of observation were required before the effect of screening was clear.

THE EFFECT OF SCREENING BY AGE: Table 9–2 summarizes the results of four experimental studies of screening in relatively young women. Despite its uncertainty, the strongest suggestion that screening women under 50 years old is valuable has come from the HIP study. A benefit of screening in this group, however, was not apparent until nearly ten years after screening began. Other studies have not yet reported follow-up for ten years or more, and positive findings in younger women have not emerged.

NONEXPERIMENTAL STUDIES

Verbeek et al (1984) used the case-control method to evaluate a program of bienniel screening with single-view mammography in Nijmegen, the Netherlands (see pages 109 to 110). The report was based on four rounds of screening. Women who participated in the program had 0.48 (0.32–1.00) times the mortality rate of breast cancer that nonparticipants had. In a subsequent analysis with 16 additional cases, the RR was 0.51 (0.26–

Table 9–2. Summary of Experimental Studies of the Effect of Screening on Breast Cancer Mortality (Women under 50 or 55 Years of Age)

Study	Age at entry (years)	Length of follow-up (years)	Percent reduction in breast cancer mortality
HIP	40–49	5	5
Shapiro et al (1988)		14	25
Two-county (Sweden)	40–49	7.9	8
Tabar et al (1989)			
Malmo	45–54	8.8	−29
Andersson et al (1988)			
Stockholm	40–49	7.4	−9
Frisell et al (1991)			

0.99). The protective effect was limited to women who were at least 50 years of age when first invited to be screened (Verbeek et al, 1985).

Collette et al (1984) used the case-control method to evaluate screening in Utrecht, the Netherlands. Screening by physical examination and xero-mammography began in 1974. Screening was done at entry, and 12, 18, and 24 months later. Women aged 50 to 64 were invited to participate. The invitation to be screened was accepted by 72%. The report was based on deaths through 1981. Participants had a breast cancer mortality rate that was 0.30 (0.13–0.70) times the rate of nonparticipants.

Palli et al (1986) used the case-control method to evaluate screening in a rural area near Florence. Screening by two-view mammography began in 1970, with the initial examinations being done between 1970 and 1981. The examinations were separated by an average interval of 2.5 years. Screening was offered to women 40 to 70 years of age. About 60% accepted the initial invitation. Participants had been offered from two to six rounds of screening. The analysis was based on breast cancer deaths in the period 1977 to 1984. Participants had a breast cancer mortality rate that was 0.53 (0.29–0.95) times the rate in nonparticipants. The data suggest a protective effect of screening in women 40 to 49, but the effect in these women was weaker than it was in older women.

Morrison et al (1988) used the follow-up method to evaluate breast cancer mortality in the Breast Cancer Detection Demonstration Project (BCDDP) in the United States. The program is described on page 46. For the first nine years after entry, breast cancer cumulative mortality in participants was 80% of the expected value. The observed to expected ratio was 0.89 for women 35 to 49 years of age at entry, 0.76 for women 50 to 59, and 0.74 for women 60 to 74. Among women screened for "routine" reasons only, without indicating a reason such as concern about breast disease, family history of breast cancer, or physician's recommendation, the observed breast cancer mortality was 62% of the expected value.

The nonexperimental studies are summarized in Table 9–3. Because breast cancer screening has been evaluated in several experiments, the findings of nonexperimental studies of the issue are relatively less important than the corresponding results would be for a disease, such as cervical cancer, for which experimental studies of screening have not been done. Nonetheless, the results are useful, and they tend to support the results of the experiments.

The case-control studies together suggest a proportional effect of screening on breast cancer mortality that is somewhat stronger than the effect suggested by the experimental studies. The nonexperimental studies, however, compare women actually screened with those who are not, while the experiments compare women assigned to be screened with those

Table 9-3. Summary of Nonexperimental Studies of the Effect of Screening on Breast Cancer Mortality

Study	Type of screening and frequency	Ages (years)	Number of subjects	Percent reduction in breast cancer mortality
Nijmegen (Verbeek et al, 1984)	Single-view mammography every two years	≥35	46 deaths 230 controls	52
Utrecht (Collette et al, 1984)	Mammography and breast palpatation at entry, 12 months, 18 months, and 24 months	50–64	46 deaths 138 controls	70
Florence (Palli et al, 1986)	Two-view mammography about every 2.5 years	40–70	57 deaths 285 controls	47
US - BCDDP (Morrison et al, 1988)	Two-view mammography and breast palpatation annually	35–74	55,053 partipants (stratified sample)	38[a]

[a]Value among women who had "routine" screening only.

not assigned to screening. Therefore, the results of the experiments are diluted by noncompliance. On the other hand, the results of the nonexperimental studies could be influenced by self-selection for screening.

Collette et al (1984) and Palli et al (1986) presented data on breast cancer mortality according to number of screening examinations taken. Such analyses are not useful because of the likelihood of healthy-screenee bias (chapter 5).

BREAST SELF-EXAMINATION

Newcomb et al (1991) described the results of a case-control study of the effectiveness of breast self-examination (BSE). The study was based on 209 women who developed advanced breast cancer and 433 controls. Advanced breast cancer was defined as TNM III or IV ("primary tumor greater than 5 cm; a tumor greater than 2 cm invading adjacent tissue other than the breast or involving fixed axillary nodes; or distant metastases"). Sixty-six percent of the cases did not have advanced disease at the time of initial diagnosis but had developed it later. Eighty-five percent of the cases had "evidence of signs and symptoms of late-stage disease in their medical records." As was appropriate, women eligible for the control series could have had early breast cancer; five such women were included in the study. Cases and controls were interviewed with respect to their practice of BSE and other relevant history. The risk of developing advanced breast cancer was found to be slightly, but not significantly, higher in women who did, compared to those who did not, report that they practiced BSE. The RR = 1.15 (0.73–1.81).

Locker et al (1989) reported the results of a case-control analysis of the relation between training in BSE and breast cancer mortality. Nearly half of the subjects were included in one of the BSE districts of the UK Trial (UK Trial of Early Detection of Cancer Group, 1988). Exposed women were defined as those who actually attended the classes in BSE to which they had been invited. Such women were reported to have reduced breast cancer mortality compared to those who did not attend; the effect was greater for women who were at least 51 years old compared to younger women. These results are very hard to interpret, however. In the UK Trial, there was no protective effect of the invitation to BSE classes. This finding, together with the protective effect of BSE training found in the case-control study, implies an unlikely relationship: that failure to attend the classes was hazardous, not simply ineffective. In addition, women were excluded from the analysis if they had breast cancer "diagnosed within 3 months of their date of invitation to education." If the training in BSE resulted in early detection, the exclusion of cases diagnosed shortly after the start of the program would create an erroneous reduction in subsequent mortality in the exposed group. Finally, it is unclear whether exposed women were more likely than unexposed women to seek other types of screening for breast cancer.

BSE at regular intervals has been recommended as a method of detecting breast cancer early (American Cancer Society, 1980). BSE has intuitive appeal, given the success of screening that includes mammography, with or without professional physical examination of the breasts. However, two studies described above showed a lack of effect of BSE (Newcomb et al, 1991; UK trial of Early Detection of Cancer Group, 1988). (The data analyzed by Locker et al (1989) overlap with one of these studies, and their results are not readily interpretable.)

It is not hard to think of reasons why these two studies could have been negative even if BSE can reduce morbidity or mortality from breast cancer (Morrison, 1991a). Compliance with the protocol and the quality of BSE are important issues. In the UK study, only about half of the women who were offered instruction in BSE actually took it, and the effect of the instruction on the practice of BSE was not described. As Newcomb et al point out, the relation between reported BSE and the actual practice of BSE was uncertain in their study. In either the Newcomb or the UK study, the BSE that was done might not have been performed well. (Newcomb et al found a nonsignificant reduced risk of advanced breast cancer among women who were judged to have practiced BSE with relatively high proficiency, but they also found a correspondingly *elevated* risk among women who practiced low-proficiency BSE.) Furthermore, the study of Newcomb et al was nonexperimental; the women selected themselves into the BSE or no-BSE categories. The results of their study could have been negatively biased by any tendency of women at relatively high risk of advanced breast cancer to practice BSE.

BSE might be effective as a primary method of screening for breast cancer in areas where the early diagnosis of breast cancer has received little emphasis and other methods of screening are not readily available. An experimental assessment of BSE is being done in the USSR (Koroltchouk et al, 1990).

BSE is a form of physical examination. The effectiveness of physical examination of the breasts by a physician or other professional health worker (without mammography) in controlling breast cancer is unknown. High-quality examinations might be easier and less costly to assure by training and monitoring a relatively small number of health professionals than by training hundreds of thousands or even millions of women in BSE. Any method of screening that is sensitive enough to detect asymptomatic cancers also results in false positives with the associated medical risks and economic costs of diagnostic evaluation that may include biopsy. The relative benefits, risks, and costs of BSE v breast examination by a professional are open questions.

The sensitivity of BSE appears low compared to other types of screening (Baines, 1989; O'Malley and Fletcher, 1987). The sensitivity probably can be improved, but the best examination techniques and methods of training are uncertain (Baines, 1988). It may be difficult to become a careful and dispassionate examiner of one's own body. The sensitivity of BSE might be expected to improve with frequent practice, but frequent BSE might also result in decreased ability to perceive a change in the breast (Baines, 1988). Unnecessarily frequent screening leads to excessive numbers of false positives. Monthly intervals for BSE should not be assumed to be optimal.

BSE has been recommended for relatively young women. The value of screening that includes mammography, however, is clearest in women who are at least 50 years old. There is substantial uncertainty as to the value of screening women in their forties. There is little information that pertains directly to the value of screening women who are less than 40, but the uncertain value of screening women 40 to 49 and the low frequency of breast cancer of women less than 40 years old suggests that screening of this group would not be rewarding. If BSE is helpful, it is likely to be most beneficial among women over 50.

BSE has been encouraged in the context of other screening in order to bring about the early treatment of cases arising between scheduled examinations (O'Malley and Fletcher, 1987). At present, women who have other types of breast cancer screening are the women who are most likely to receive encouragement and instruction in BSE. If BSE can be effective, these are the women who are least likely to benefit from the practice. The low prevalence of detectable asymptomatic cases shortly after a screening examination and the relatively low sensitivity of BSE together imply that few if any cases would be found early enough to gain much therapeutic advantage. In addition, the ratio of false positives to true positives would probably be high. As screening technology improves, the relative frequency of interval cases, and any benefit of BSE for women screened by other means, will decrease further.

Many breast cancers are brought to medical attention by the affected women themselves. This might be taken as an argument to support BSE, but the process of perceiving symptoms and seeking care for them should be distinguished from a disease-control *policy* of BSE. The results described above provide no support for the use of BSE in screening.

CONCLUSIONS

The early detection and treatment of breast cancer based on screening that includes mammography reduces mortality from the disease. Every study of this relation has been positive, with one exception: the Malmo trial. That study was relatively small and a relatively high fraction of the control group had mammography.

The types of screening that have been shown to be effective are two-view mammography and physical examination combined, and single-view or two-view mammography alone. The effect of screening by physical examination alone has not been studied. There is no direct evidence that self-examination reduces mortality from breast cancer.

The schedules of screening that have been shown to be effective have varied from approximately yearly (two-view mammography and physical examination together) to approximately every 33 months (single-view mammography alone).

The value of screening women 50 to 74 years of age is clear. The value of screening women 40 to 49 is less certain. If there is a reduction in mortality in this group, it probably takes longer to appear than it does in older women. Almost no information is available on the value of screening women under 40 with present methods. Screening normal-risk women under 40 is likely to be unrewarding because of the infrequency of breast cancer.

Although there is little direct evidence on the value of screening at ages older than 74, the findings in women 60 to 74 imply that screening would be effective among women over 74 in reducing deaths from breast cancer. Assuming that screening is effective in this group, however, there are additional important influences on the benefit of screening in the old. These are the delay before the effect of screening appears, the high mortality from causes other than breast cancer, and the self-selection of healthy persons, who have relatively long life expectancies, into screening programs. The last of these influences tends to counterbalance the other two, but the effect of the three together is unclear. Thus, the age at which the benefit of screening would become too small to be useful is unknown.

The effect of screening, at least in women 50 to 74 years old, is large enough to justify organized efforts at early detection as a control measure for breast cancer. The available evidence justifies screening at intervals from 12 to 33 months, by use of mammography alone or together with physical examination. Although the effect of screening is substantial, breast cancer will continue to be an important problem given present methods of detection and treatment.

The studies that have been done were, of necessity, of relatively short duration. There is considerable uncertainty in using the results of these studies to estimate the effects of a screening policy that spans a large part of adult life. For example, the contributions of initial (prevalence) cases v later (incidence) cases to reductions in mortality are not known, but the information could influence long-term screening policy. If prevalence cases account for a disproportionately large contribution to reduction in mortality, screening might not have to be done especially frequently.

Despite improvements in mammography, the reductions in mortality observed in recent experimental studies have been no larger—and some have been smaller—than the reduction observed in the HIP study. Other than chance variation, possible reasons for the lack of continuing improvement in the results of studies include the following: (a) less frequent screening in recent studies than in early studies; (b) irrelevance of recent improvements in mammography to the reduction in mortality—that is, most reduction in mortality is attributable to tumors that are easy to see and would be found even with relatively crude mammography; (c) lack of screening by physical examination; (d) use of single-view mammography; (e) increasingly early detection of breast cancer with the passage of time as a result of background screening; (f) improvements in the treatment of breast cancer that have made screening less important in the control of the disease than was the case 10 or 20 years ago. These explanations of the trend of results are speculative; none has been shown to be correct.

A "baseline" mammogram has been recommended for relatively young (eg, 35- to 40-year-old) women (American Cancer Society's National Task Force on Breast Cancer Control, 1982). The sensitivity of a subsequent mammogram might be increased if a baseline mammogram makes it easier to identify changes in breast structure caused by a small cancer, but it is not obvious that such an enhancement of sensitivity would increase the benefit of screening very much. It seems unlikely that the specificity of screening would be enhanced by baseline mammography except for cases in which a suspicious image in a subsequent mammogram corresponded to an image that had been overlooked in the baseline mammogram. The value of baseline mammography has not been addressed in any of the studies that have provided the foundation for other aspects of screening policy for breast cancer. It is difficult to imagine the design of a practical study that would shed light on this issue, especially in view of the uncertain effectiveness of any type of breast cancer screening for women in their forties. Furthermore, a baseline mammogram is also a screening mammogram. There is not likely to be much disease-control value in screening women under 40, but such screening inevitably has costs and adverse effects such as biopsies related to false positives. A policy of baseline mammography is not advisable unless its value can be shown to justify its costs and risks.

10 Cardiovascular Disease

Cardiovascular disease (CVD) is the leading cause of death in many countries and methods of controlling CVD are needed. Intensive research on the epidemiology of CVD began in the 1940s and 1950s with a number of follow-up studies. The most important risk factors for CVD to be discovered in these studies were cigarette smoking, hypertension, and high serum cholesterol (Pooling Project Research Group, 1978). Additional risk factors for CVD include obesity, lack of exercise, and excessive dietary salt and fat (Fraser, 1986).

One general approach to the control of CVD is through preventive measures such as population recommendations regarding smoking cessation, weight loss, exercise, and changes in the content of the diet. CVD might also be controlled by screening in order to identify persons who have conditions such as high blood pressure or high serum cholesterol but no symptoms of CVD. These persons can be offered drug treatment, intensive dietary counseling, or another intervention to slow the progress of the disease. The major components of CVD are ischemic heart disease (including myocardial infarction and sudden death) and cerebrovascular disease (including thrombotic and hemorrhagic stroke). A successful screening program will reduce disability or death from one or both of these sources.

Most evidence related to screening for CVD is provided by experimental studies that concerned the value of treatment among persons with confirmed positive screening tests for hypertension or hypercholesterolemia; persons with negative tests were not kept under observation. As pointed out in chapter 4 (pages 76 to 77), this approach provides less information on the value of screening as a means of disease control than studies, such as those on breast cancer, in which entire screened and unscreened populations are compared. Nonetheless, some information on the disease control value of screening for CVD can be derived from the studies that have been done.

This chapter begins with a review of the methods and results of studies in which subjects were identified by screening, and in which the effect of early treatment on death from CVD can be related to the number of persons screened. The studies are grouped into those on hypertension, hypercholesterolemia, or multiple factors. Then the information is interpreted with respect to the value of screening as a control measure for CVD.

The studies are summarized in Table 10–1, which gives the numbers of subjects screened, the proportions of screenees randomized to one of the treatments, the periods of follow-up, and the treated-control differences in deaths from ischemic heart disease, cerebrovascular disease, and all cardiovascular disease. The types of events included in these categories vary according to the information available for each study. For example, deaths from ischemic heart disease might correspond to fatal coronary events (Medical Research Council Working Party, 1985) or to deaths from myocardial infarction plus other ischemic heart disease (Hypertension Detection and Follow-up Program Cooperative Group, 1979). Deaths from all cardiovascular disease might simply be the sum of deaths from ischemic heart disease and cerebrovascular disease (Management Committee, 1980), or the category might include additional entities such as hypertensive heart disease (Hypertension Detection and Follow-up Program Cooperative Group, 1979) or peripheral vascular disease (Lipid Research Clinics Program, 1984).

STUDIES ON HYPERTENSION

Methods and Results

The value of the medical treatment of hypertension in the clinical setting is well established (Veterans Administration Cooperative Study Group on Antihypertensive Agents, 1967, 1970). In contrast to the clinical studies, persons with symptomatic or previously diagnosed disease were not eligible for the studies described below.

HYPERTENSION DETECTION AND FOLLOW-UP PROGRAM (HDFP)(1979): Men and women were "recruited by population-based screening of 158,906 people aged 30 to 69 years. . . ." The main criterion of eligibility was a diastolic blood pressure $\geq$ 90mm. A total of 10,940 subjects were randomized to Stepped Care, a standardized and carefully monitored treatment program

Table 10–1. Summary of Experimental Studies of Treatment of Hypertension or Hypercholesterolemia among Subjects Identified by Screening

Study	Number screened	Proportion of screenees randomized	Years of follow-up	Reduction in deaths per number screened times 10^5		
				Ischemic heart disease	Cerebrovascular disease	All cardiovascular disease
Hypertension						
Hypertension Detection and Follow-up Program (1979)	158,906	.069	5	21.4[a] (17)[b]	28.9 (23)	56.6 (45)
Australian Therapeutic Trial in Mild Hypertension (Management Committee, 1980)	104,171	.033	4	11.5 (6)	5.8 (3)	17.3 (9)
Oslo (Helgeland, 1980)	16,200	.049	5.5	−49.4 (−4)	24.7 (2)	0.0 (0)
Medical Research Council Trial (1985)	515,000	.034	4.9	−3.5 (−9)	3.5 (9)	1.9 (5)
Hypercholesterolemia						
Clofibrate (Committee of Principal Investigators, 1978)	52,519	.202	13.2	−95.2 (−25)	−57.1 (−15)	−114.2 (−30)
Lipid Research Clinics Program (1984)	480,000	.008	7.4	5.0 (12)	0.0 (0)	4.2 (10)
Helsinki Heart Study (1987)	18,966	.215	5	52.7 (5)	−21.1 (−2)	5.3 (1)
Multifactor						
Oslo (Hjermann et al, 1981)	16,202	.076	5	98.8 (8)	−12.3 (−1)	86.4 (7)
Multiple Risk Factor Intervention Trial (1982, 1990)	361,662	.036	10.5	13.3 (24)	1.7 (3)	19.9 (36)

[a] These values assume that all screen-detected cases were assigned to the special treatment group.
[b] The control-treated number of deaths is given in parentheses.

designed "to achieve and maintain reduction of [blood pressure] to or below set goals," or to Referred Care, that is, "referred to their usual sources of care, with special referral efforts for those with more severe hypertension or organ damage." Subjects were followed up for five years. The number of deaths from all causes was 349 for Stepped Care v 419 for Referred Care. The difference in favor of Stepped Care appeared as early as the first year of follow-up. The largest difference, 86 v 111, occurred in the fourth year. The numbers of deaths in the fifth year were equal (at 91). The cause-specific numbers of deaths were 195 v 240 for all cardiovascular diseases, 29 v 52 for cerebrovascular diseases, 51 v 69 for myocardial infarction, and 154 v 179 for all noncardiovascular causes.

AUSTRALIAN TRIAL (Management Committee, 1980): There were 104,171 men and women volunteers aged 30 to 69 years who were screened. To be eligible for randomization, the diastolic blood pressure had to be 95 to 109mm and the systolic blood pressure <200mm. The "trial population" numbered 3,427 (3.3% of screened subjects). Participants were randomized to active treatment or placebo. Both groups were reexamined at regular intervals. If a sustained rise in blood pressure above the eligibility level was observed, "definitive" treatment was given. In the course of the trial, this was done for 198 in the placebo group and 4 in the treatment group. The average period of follow-up was four years. The total number of cases of ischemic heart disease was 98 in the treatment group and 109 in the placebo group. There were 5 v 11 fatal cases, 28 v 22 nonfatal myocardial infarctions, and 65 v 76 other nonfatal cases. There were 17 v 31 cerebrovascular events: 3 v 6 fatal events, 10 v 16 nonfatal strokes, and 4 v 9 cases of transient cerebral ischemic attack. There were 25 deaths from all causes in the treated group v 35 in the placebo group. The effect of treatment did not vary much with age or sex.

THE OSLO STUDY OF MILD HYPERTENSION (Helgeland, 1980): All Oslo men aged 40 to 49 years were invited for screening and 16,200 (65%) accepted. Men whose systolic blood pressure was 150 to 179mm and diastolic blood pressure <110mm (or systolic pressure <150mm but diastolic pressure 95 to 109mm) were eligible. There were 785 men randomized to active treatment or a control group (no placebo). Both groups were monitored as the study progressed. If blood pressure increased to ≥180mm systolic or ≥110mm diastolic, active treatment was given. This was done for 17% of controls. The average period of follow-up was 66 months (range 60 to 78 months). There were 6 "coronary deaths" in the treated group v 2 in the control group. There were 0 v 4 "noncoronary vascular deaths," and

10 *v* 9 total deaths. There were 25 *v* 34 "total cardiovascular events"; 20 *v* 13 "coronary events"; 0 *v* 7 "cerebrovascular events" including 0 *v* 2 fatal subarachnoid hemorrhages; and 5 *v* 14 "other [cardiovascular] events."

MEDICAL RESEARCH COUNCIL (MRC) TRIAL OF TREATMENT OF MILD HYPERTENSION (1985): Men and women aged 35 to 64 years were identified by use of registers of group practices in England, Scotland, and Wales. Of 695,000 persons invited to be screened, 515,000 (74%) accepted. Of those screened, 20,600 were determined to be eligible, based on entry blood pressure (diastolic 90 to 109mm, systolic <200mm). Of those eligible, 16,410 (nearly 80%) agreed to participate. Another 944 participants were recruited elsewhere, for a total of 17,354 participants. These were randomized into three groups: a placebo group and two active treatments of hypertension (bendrofluazide or propanolol). For those on active treatment, additional drugs were used if the assigned drug did not have a sufficient effect on the blood pressure. If, in the course of the study, the blood pressures of control subjects exceeded specified levels, active treatment was begun. Subjects were followed up for an average of 4.9 years. Sixty strokes occurred in the treated group *v* 109 in the placebo group (18 *v* 27 fatal strokes). There were 222 "coronary events" in the treated group and 234 in the placebo group (106 *v* 97 fatal coronary events). There were 286 "all cardiovascular events" in the treated group *v* 352 in the placebo group, 134 *v* 139 "all cardiovascular deaths," and 248 total deaths in the treated group *v* 253 in the placebo group. There were no convincing differences in the efficacy of treatment for men *v* women.

KAISER STUDY (Friedman et al, 1986): The methods and results of the Kaiser Health Plan study of multiphasic screening are described on pages 87 to 90. This is the only study reviewed in this chapter in which mortality can be compared directly between groups assigned, or not assigned, to a screening program. Mortality from ischemic heart disease was the same in the study and control groups. Mortality from "hypertension, hypertensive heart disease, and hemorrhagic stroke preceded by hypertension" was lower in the study than in the control group. It is likely, however, that the latter difference was the result of more intensive treatment in the study than the control group of previously diagnosed hypertensives, rather than the early detection and treatment of new cases. There was virtually no difference between the groups in mortality from hypertension and related conditions among persons not known to be hypertensive before enrollment (Dales et al, 1979).

Comments

In each of the four studies of the treatment of screen-detected hypertension alone, the number of deaths from cerebrovascular disease was lower in the special treatment group compared to the control group. Except for the HDFP, however, the differences were small. Mortality from ischemic heart disease was reduced in the special treatment group in two of the studies, but increased in the other two. The only large reduction in total CVD deaths was found in the HDFP. In some of the studies, the incidence of nonfatal stroke was substantially lower in the special treatment group compared to the control group. This difference may imply an important effect of screening on disability. Continued follow-up would be needed to determine the relation of this difference to a subsequent difference in mortality.

The methods of the HDFP differed from the other studies in two important respects (Fries, 1982). First, members of the Referred Care group who developed severe hypertension after their initial referral might not have been treated quickly or aggressively. In the other studies, control subjects were monitored periodically and those who developed severe hypertension were treated. If the early detection and treatment of hypertension is effective, the difference in protocol implies that the HDFP would be expected to show a larger difference in mortality between the groups than would the other studies.

Second, the HDFP compared intensive to less intensive care, rather than a particular treatment to a placebo as in the other studies. Subjects assigned to the Stepped Care regimen might have had generally better medical care than the subjects assigned to Referred Care. Support for this idea is provided by the observation of lower mortality from noncardiovascular causes in the Stepped Care compared to the Referred Care group. Thus, some of the difference in cardiovascular mortality between the groups might be attributable to generally better care given to the Stepped Care group rather than to specific antihypertensive treatment. A difference in *non*cardiovascular mortality as a result of nonspecific differences between the Stepped Care and Referred Care regimens would be very small in relation to all noncardiovascular mortality in the entire screened population.

The lack of reported effect of screening on mortality related to hypertension in the Kaiser study may seem puzzling, but there are at least two explanations for it. First, there was only a modest difference in the proportions of subjects screened at least once in the test group (84%) compared to the control group (64%). As suggested below, there might be little additional benefit of frequent, compared to infrequent, screening for hypertension. If so, the similarity of exposure would greatly reduce any difference in mortality between the groups. Second, the number of persons studied was relatively small. Even with 16 years of follow-up, few deaths related to hypertension would be expected among subjects not known to have the condition at entry. Thus, the power of the study was low.

STUDIES ON HYPERCHOLESTEROLEMIA

Methods and Results

Blood levels of cholesterol and other lipids may be changed by either diet or drugs. In the studies described in this section, drugs were used to reduce cholesterol levels. As with the studies of hypertension, symptomatic persons were not eligible. Dietary modification was used in the multifactorial studies that are described subsequently. The value of dietary modification to control CVD also has been investigated in persons not previously selected according to blood lipid levels. Such studies are not reviewed here because they are considered to be studies of prevention rather than screening.

CLOFIBRATE TRIAL (Committee of Principal Investigators, 1978, 1984): There were 52,519 men aged 30 to 59 years who were screened. The experiment was based on 10,627 men who were in the upper third of the distribution of serum cholesterol level at initial screening. The participants were assigned at random to treatment with Clofibrate (a cholesterol-lowering drug) or placebo. The period of intervention averaged 5.3 years. During this period there were 36 deaths from fatal ischemic heart disease in the treated group v 34 in the control group, and 7 v 4 deaths from stroke. There were 131 v 174 nonfatal myocardial infarctions. There were 128 v 87 deaths from all causes combined. There were 42 v 25 deaths from cancer, a trend that was apparent for a number of specific sites. The men were followed for an average of 7.9 years after the intervention ended. Over the entire period of observation (an average of 13.2 years) there were 308 v 283 deaths from ischemic heart disease, 62 v 47 deaths from stroke, 404 v 374 deaths from ischemic heart disease, stroke, and other circulatory disease combined, 206 v 197 deaths from cancer, and 720 v 650 deaths from all causes.

LIPID RESEARCH CLINICS TRIAL (1984): There were 480,000 male volunteers aged 35 to 59 years who were screened. Subjects were eligible if the plasma cholesterol level was $\geq$ 265 mg/dl and the low-density lipoprotein cholesterol level was $\geq$ 190 mg/dl. Subjects were excluded for an average triglyceride level > 300 mg/dl, type III hyperlipoproteinemia, as well as hypertension or evidence of ischemic heart disease. The study was based on 3,806 men. All were instructed in a moderate cholesterol-lowering diet. The men were randomly assigned to one of two groups: treatment with cholestyramine (a cholesterol-lowering drug) or placebo. The men were followed for an average of 7.4 years (range, 7–10). There were 32 "definite or suspect" coronary heart disease deaths in the treated group v 44 in the placebo group. Of these, there were 30 v 38 "definite" coronary heart disease deaths. There were 2 v 2 deaths from cerebrovascular disease. There were 37 v 47 deaths from all cardiovascular causes. There were 68 v 71 deaths from all causes. There were 195 v 225 "definite or suspect nonfatal myocardial infarctions," of which 130 v 158 were "definite." There were 18 v 22 "definite or suspect" cases of transient cerebral ischemic attack and 17 v 14 cases of "definite or suspect atherothrombotic brain infarction." The beneficial effect of treatment on the incidence of ischemic heart disease began to appear after about two years of follow-up. The size of the cumulative treated-placebo difference generally increased subsequently.

HELSINKI HEART STUDY (Frick et al, 1987): There were 23,531 male civil service or industrial employees aged 40 to 55 who were identified as eligible for screening. Of these, 18,966 (80.6%) agreed to be screened. Men eligible to be randomized had a non-high-density lipoprotein cholesterol level $\geq$ 200 mg/dl (5.2 mmol/l) at each of two examinations. There were 4,081 men who met the eligibility criteria and who agreed to be randomized; these were assigned to treatment with gemfibrozil or placebo. The men were followed for five years. There were 14 deaths from ischemic heart disease among the men assigned to gemfibrozil v 19 among those assigned to placebo. There were 1 v 3 deaths from ischemic cerebral infarction and 5 v 1 deaths from intracranial hemorrhage. There were 22 v 23 deaths from all cardiovascular causes. There were 45 v 42 deaths from all causes. There were 45 definite nonfatal myocardial infarctions in the gemfibrozil group v 71 in the placebo group. There were more gastrointestinal operations in the gemfibrozil group than there were in the placebo group (81 v 53).

Comments

The treatment of hypercholesterolemia alone has not been clearly related to the reduction of mortality from ischemic heart disease in screened populations. Although decreases in such deaths were observed among treated subjects in the Lipid Research Clinics study and the Helsinki Heart Study, there was an increase in ischemic heart disease deaths observed in the Clofibrate trial. There was no evidence that the treatment of hypercholesterolemia reduced mortality from cerebrovascular disease. There were small or moderate reductions in nonfatal myocardial infarction among the treated subjects in each of the three studies. In the Clofibrate trial, the study group had a *higher* death rate from all causes than the control group did. In the other studies, all cause mortality was similar in study and control groups.

MULTIFACTOR STUDIES

Methods and Results

Studies have been done in which asymptomatic subjects were identified for intervention in relation to two or more risk factors for CVD. Each study involved screening for and treatment of at least hypertension or hypercholesterolemia.

OSLO STUDY (Hjermann et al, 1981): All Oslo men aged 40 to 49 years of age were invited for screening and 16,202 (65%) accepted. The men selected for study had an average serum cholesterol level of 290 to 380 mg/dl, "coronary risk scores (based on cholesterol levels, smoking habits and blood pressure) in the upper quartile," and average systolic blood pressure <150mm. Men were excluded for diabetes, a serum cholesterol level ≥ 380 mg/dl, or being on a lipid-lowering diet. There were 1,232 men randomized. Men in the intervention group received dietary counseling intended to lower the blood lipids, and were advised to stop smoking, if relevant. Both the intervention and control groups were followed up for five years. There were 8 CVD deaths in the intervention group *v* 15 in the control group. Of these, 3 *v* 11 were "sudden coronary" deaths, 3 *v* 2 were fatal myocardial infarction, and 2 *v* 1 were fatal stroke. There were 16 *v* 24 deaths from all causes. There were 13 *v* 22 nonfatal myocardial infarctions, 1 *v* 2 nonfatal strokes, and 22 *v* 39 "total cardiovascular events" (fatal and nonfatal).

MULTIPLE RISK FACTOR INTERVENTION TRIAL (MRFIT) (1982, 1990): There were 361,662 male volunteers aged 35 to 57 years who were screened. Potentially eligible subjects had levels of serum cholesterol or diastolic blood pressure, or a history of cigarette smoking, that placed them in the upper 15% or 10% of risk of coronary heart disease (as based on data from the Framingham study). Exclusion criteria included evidence of myocardial infarction, serum cholesterol ≥ 350 mg/dl, diastolic blood pressure ≥115mm, and extreme obesity. There were 12,866 men randomized to Special Intervention or Usual Care. The Special Intervention included dietary counseling aimed at reduction of blood lipid levels, reduction of caloric intake for overweight men, a smoking cessation program, and treatment of hypertension. The duration of intervention was six to eight years depending on the time of enrollment. During this period (an average of 6.9 years of observation per subject) the intervention had little apparent effect; there were 110 coronary heart disease deaths in the Special Intervention group v 117 in the Usual Care group, 143 v 144 total cardiovascular disease deaths, 123 v 118 noncardiovascular deaths, and 266 v 262 total deaths. With continuing observation, however, some differences in outcome between the two groups were seen. During the 3.8 years after the end of the intervention, there were 92 v 109 coronary heart disease deaths, 123 v 146 total cardiovascular disease deaths, 107 v 129 noncardiovascular disease deaths, and 230 v 275 total deaths. Over the entire observation period there were 106 v 140 deaths from myocardial infarction and 96 v 86 deaths from other ischemic heart disease. There were 20 v 23 deaths from cerebrovascular disease and 266 v 290 deaths from all CVD. In the first 6.9 years of observation, there were 294 v 323 nonfatal myocardial infarctions, and 1,266 v 1,502 other nonfatal cardiovascular events.

Comments

In both multifactorial studies, mortality attributable to all CVD was lower in the special treatment group than in the control group. The difference was almost entirely limited to ischemic heart disease. The reduction in mortality per number screened in the Oslo study was much larger than that in the MRFIT study, but the source of the disparity is not obvious. The methods of the two studies differed in many respects. Furthermore, the Oslo study was relatively small. The reduction of mortality from ischemic heart disease per number screened in the MRFIT study was less than that in the HDFP and similar to that in the Australian trial. The latter two studies concerned only hypertension. Both multifactorial studies included dietary modification to reduce serum cholesterol. The designs of the studies, however, make it difficult to separate the effects of the individual interventions.

The MRFIT study was the most comprehensive effort to date at evaluating the control of CVD by screening and treatment of the persons found to be at high risk. The effect of the special program on cardiovascular mortality was relatively small. Compliance with the assigned protocol, however, was imperfect. In particular, the knowledge of being at high risk appears to have had a strong effect on the distribution of risk factors among members of the Usual Care group. Within a year of the start of the study, the mean diastolic blood pressures of both the Special Intervention and Usual Care groups were less than 90mm and were separated by only a few mm. Likewise, the mean blood cholesterol levels of the two groups a year after the start were below 250 mg/dl and were separated by less than 10 mg/dl. Thus, the program might be more effective than it appeared.

Both multifactorial studies included smoking-cessation programs. As with the treatments of hypertension and hypercholesterolemia, the effects of the smoking-cessation programs are not readily disentangled from the other interventions in the two studies. The benefits of not smoking so clearly outweigh the costs that there is no reason not to advocate smoking cessation. Furthermore, smokers know who they are without any special testing, and it is in their own interests to quit irrespective of their blood pressure or cholesterol levels. Smoking cessation is more appropriately considered as prevention than as early detection and treatment.

INTERPRETATION

In the experiments summarized in Table 10–1, screening was used to find eligible subjects, but those screened negative were not followed up. Therefore, the results of these studies provide no direct indication of the proportion of the total mortality from a disease that might be reduced by a screening program. On the other hand, the reduction in mortality brought about by treatment can be related to the number of persons screened. The values shown in the last three columns of Table 10–1 assume that *all* screen-detected cases (instead of half) were assigned to the special treatment group so that the results are readily compared with findings in studies of cancer screening.

Compared to screening for breast cancer, the effect of screening for CVD on mortality has generally appeared to be small in relation to the number of people screened. In the HIP study, the screened group experienced 23 fewer deaths from breast cancer over the first five years of the study. In relation to the 20,000 women who were actually screened, the reduction in cumulative mortality from breast cancer was 115 per 100,000. The largest reduction in CVD deaths per number screened—a benefit numerically comparable to that found in the HIP study—was seen in the Oslo multifactorial study. This study was relatively small, however. In the HDFP, the most strongly positive of the large studies, the reduction in cumulative mortality from stroke among the screened persons was only about one-quarter of the benefit seen in the HIP study, and the reduction in all CVD deaths was about one-half of that value. Much smaller benefits were observed in most of the remaining studies. It should be noted that all experimental studies of screening for breast cancer, including the HIP, have used repeated screening. The extents to which the first, v subsequent, examinations contributed to the observed reductions in mortality are unknown.

Death from various manifestations of CVD is much more common than is death from breast cancer. Therefore, it may be inferred that only a small *proportional* reduction in CVD mortality is brought about by any of the programs described. This reduction is relatively small because most deaths from CVD occur in the large segment of the population that has "normal" levels of blood pressure or serum cholesterol; the death rate in this group would not be affected by screening (Rose, 1987). In the Pooling Project (The Pooling Project Research Group, 1978), for example, only one-third of the stroke deaths in men observed over ten years occurred in those whose starting diastolic blood pressure was $\geq$ 95mm. Even if screening could reduce stroke deaths in the latter group by 50%, the proportional benefit to the entire population would be only a one-sixth reduction.

In most of the studies of hypertension and in some studies of hypercholesterolemia, potential subjects identified by screening were excluded for very high, as well as for low, values. (In the HDFP, medical follow-up was ensured for Referred Care subjects with diastolic blood pressure $\geq$ 115 mm.) Presumably, the subjects with very high blood pressure or serum cholesterol were to be treated regardless of initial assignment. The exclusion of these patients, however, makes it difficult to determine the effect of treating *all* persons who meet a given screening or diagnostic cut-off level. The greatest short-term effect of treating hypertension has been observed among subjects with the highest entry levels of blood pressure (Veterans Administration Cooperative Study Group on Antihypertensive Agents, 1967, 1970, 1972). Men with especially high levels of blood pressure were excluded from most studies based on screened subjects, but if such subjects had been included, the apparent benefit of screening might have been greater. On the other hand, subjects in the studies done in clinical settings may also have had more to gain in the short term from treatment than did subjects in the studies on screened groups, for a given starting level of blood pressure. This would be true if treatment is disproportionately effective among persons with symptoms or other evidence of advanced disease who would have been excluded from the screening studies in any event.

The periods of follow-up in most of the studies were five to seven years. This is a fairly short time in which to measure the effect of the early detection and treatment of a chronic disease. A period of this length may be sufficient to indicate whether a beneficial effect of early treatment on the incidence of ischemic heart disease or cerebrovascular disease is likely to exist, but an effect on mortality may be difficult to perceive. The recent positive results on mortality in the MRFIT study (The Multiple Risk Factor Intervention Trial Research Group, 1990), and the comparatively large effects of treatment on incidence in several of the studies, suggest the potential value of long-term observations. A five- to seven-year follow-up period also is too brief to distinguish short-term postponement of incidence of, or death from, CVD v cures or long-term postponement of these events. Furthermore, such a period is too brief to be confident about the extent of adverse effects of treatment. Finally, a five- to seven-year period is almost certainly too short to suggest the size of the entire cumulative effect of a treatment that continues indefinitely. If the effects of early treatment that have been observed do reflect long-term benefits, the public health value of screening is almost certainly greater than that suggested by the published studies.

Measures of CVD incidence have been used as outcomes in addition to CVD mortality. Incident cases have the statistical advantages of occurring more frequently and sooner than deaths. Because they are acute and symptomatic, myocardial infarction and stroke, including nonfatal cases, may appear to be satisfactory indicators of advanced morbidity for evaluating early detection and treatment. In general, however, myocardial infarction is not as closely associated with rapid death as symptomatic metastatic cancer is. Mortality is high shortly after a myocardial infarction, but a high fraction of patients with myocardial infarction survive long after diagnosis, many suffering little significant disability (British Medical Journal, 1979; Gentry, 1979; Kuller, 1979). Therefore it is possible that the early treatment of CVD as found by screening reduces the incidence of relatively mild, but not severe, myocardial infarction. There are, furthermore, "silent" myocardial infarctions. They may confuse the interpretation of the apparent relation between screening and morbidity, depending on the effect that early treatment has on "silent" myocardial infarction and on the mortality of the persons affected. Broadly similar problems pertain to the interpretation of nonfatal strokes. It is likely, however, that the average degree of disability and the average case fatality are higher after a stroke than after a myocardial infarction.

The evaluation of screening for CVD is hampered by its heterogeneity. Several tests and treatments must be studied in relation to different diagnostic entities. The type of early treatment recommended depends on which screening test is positive. Treatments for hypertension are likely to have different effects on ischemic heart disease and cerebrovascular disease than are treatments for hypercholesterolemia. The Clofibrate study suggested that lipid-lowering treatment may have serious side effects not obviously related to the vascular system. Thus, interventions have been related to several causes of death. Inevitably, the pattern of associations has varied from study to study.

Because of uncertainty as to the specific causes of death that may be favorably or unfavorably affected by a given intervention, the results should be analyzed in relation to broad categories of cause of death. Mortality from all causes combined provides a comprehensive measure of the value of the intervention. All-cause mortality is a relatively insensitive measure for evaluating the effect of the treatment on a specific cause of death because of the effect of random fluctuations in causes of death not related to the treatment. In general, however, the treated-control differences in all-cause mortality are similar to the differences in CVD mortality. The excess all-cause mortality in the Clofibrate study was mentioned previously. The all-cause mortality is reduced more than the CVD mortality in the HDFP; this discrepancy was discussed in the section on studies of hypertension.

Medical treatments for hypertension or hypercholesterolemia are associated with various adverse effects (Joint National Committee on Detection, Evaluation, and Treatment of High Blood Pressure, 1984; Tikkanen and Nikkila, 1987). Mild side effects may discourage long-term compliance, diminishing the value of screening, while other side effects may be serious and even fatal. As shown by the proportions of screenees randomized (Table 10–1), substantial proportions of those screened may be treated. It is important not to expose large numbers of persons unnecessarily to the risks (and costs) of treatment for hypertension. Information on side effects is incomplete because the periods of observation have been short in most of the reported studies.

Virtually no information is available on the benefit of screening according to age, sex, or race. Although some studies have provided results of treatment for such subgroups, the results were not related to the corresponding numbers of persons screened.

CONCLUSIONS

On balance, the available evidence provides modest support for screening for hypertension and only slight support for screening for hypercholesterolemia in the control of CVD. Even if screening is accepted as valuable, the designs of the studies that have been done seriously limit the available information on which to base specific screening recommendations. Many fundamental questions need better answers than are available now.

How should hypertension and hypercholesterolemia be defined diagnostically? Should the definitions depend on age or sex? What types of screening measurements should be made? What cut-off levels should be used? Anxiety or fear, and metabolic or physiologic fluctuations, may affect the sensitivity and specificity of screening (Armitage et al, 1966). These influences should be understood and accommodated in the design of screening procedures.

What are appropriate screening schedules? At what age should screening begin? How often should screening be done subsequently? Should screening schedules vary by sex, race, or other personal characteristics?

Information on which to base screening schedules may be derived directly from studies that compare the effects of different schedules. Given that such comparative data are not available, screening schedules could be developed from knowledge of sensitivities of screening and the natural histories of hypertension and hypercholesterolemia. The necessary information includes the rates at which these conditions arise in previously normal people, the rates at which newly-established hypertension or hypercholesterolemia then progress to cause death or serious illness, and the relation of progression to the initial levels and to age and sex. It would also be necessary to know the long-term effects of treatment on both mortality and serious morbidity such as strokes. Nearly all studies of the treatment of screen-detected hypertension or hypercholesterolemia were ended too soon.

Although some recommendations for frequent screening have been made, it has been found that a given individual tends to maintain a position within a population distribution of blood pressure or serum cholesterol (Fraser, 1986). Such "tracking" implies that the rates at which persons become newly hypertensive or hypercholesterolemic may be low. Frequent screening may result in large numbers of false positives but only small numbers of new true positive cases that would benefit from treatment.

Finally, both blood pressure and serum cholesterol can be reduced by nonmedical means. What are the relative costs and benefits of screening v population recommendations regarding reductions in dietary salt and fat, weight reduction, and exercise, irrespective of blood pressure or serum cholesterol level? Some obvious advantages of the latter approach are inclusion of persons with normal levels of blood pressure and cholesterol, in whom most CVD occurs; avoidance of the costs of screening; and avoidance of the adverse effects of medications. CVD mortality has fallen sharply in the United States during the past two decades; smaller decreases have been noted in other areas (Fraser, 1986). The causes of the trends are uncertain, but population-wide changes in smoking, diet, and exercise patterns are plausible explanations.

11   Cancer of the Cervix

Cancer of the cervix is the epitome of a disease for which screening is attractive. There is a period of years or even decades during which preclinical disease can be detected (Boyes et al, 1982; Task force, 1976). Furthermore, most screen-detected cervical cancer is in situ, which implies that treatment is likely to cure the disease. Cytologic screening for cancer of the cervix became an accepted part of medical practice before the need for mortality-based experimentation was widely recognized. Because it does not now seem possible to carry out experimental studies, screening recommendations must be based entirely on evidence assembled by nonexperimental methods.

Cervical cancer screening has been related to mortality from the disease primarily by use of geographic and temporal correlations. This chapter begins with a summary of these studies and an interpretation of the results. The next section concerns case-control studies of screening for cervical cancer. The studies are reviewed and the methodological issues that they raise are discussed. Next, the results of an indirect approach to formulating screening policy are reviewed. This approach makes use of the time trend in the incidence rate of invasive cervical cancer in negatively screened women. Finally, some general conclusions are given as to the efficacy of screening for cervical cancer and screening policy for the disease.

CORRELATION STUDIES

The most useful data on the effectiveness of screening for cancer of the cervix are drawn from five Nordic countries. The data are summarized in Table 11–1. The information is especially valuable because trends in cer-

Table 11-1. Screening and Trends in Mortality from Cervical Cancer in Nordic Countries

Country	Screening Interval in years	Screening Rank[a]	Cervical cancer mortality rate[b] 1963–1967	Cervical cancer mortality rate[b] 1978–1982	Mortality rate difference[c]	Percentage reduction in mortality
Denmark	3	2 (1980)	25.3	17.6	7.7	30
Finland	5	4 (1970)	51.4	23.4	28.0	54
Iceland	2–3	5 (1969)	70.4	18.8	51.5	73
Norway	2–3	1 (1960)	51.9	47.8	4.1	8
Sweden	4	3 (1973)	51.2	32.3	18.9	37

Source: Based on Laara et al (1987).

[a] The rank reflects the proportion of women who were covered by and attended screening programs; the lowest rank corresponds to the smallest proportion screened. The year in which the respective coverage was achieved is given in parentheses.

[b] Mean of age-specific numbers of deaths per 100,000 PY among women 30 to 69 years of age.

[c] Difference in mortality rate from 1963–1967 to 1978–1982.

vical cancer mortality can be related to specific screening policies as well as to the level of participation.

DENMARK (Laara et al, 1987; Lynge, 1983): Screening programs have been organized in several counties of Denmark. The first began in 1962, and the most recent began in 1981. The recommendations with respect to age groups and frequencies of screening have differed somewhat among the programs, as has the screening technique (self-administered smears in some areas; professional screening in others). Women 30 to 50 years old have been included in every program. The average interval between invitations to be screened is approximately three years. As of 1980, 40% of the population was covered by a screening program, and about 80% of women invited to screening attended. Mortality from cervical cancer rose sharply from 1953–1955 to 1956–1958 and then fell slightly. From 1963–1967 to 1978–1982 the rate decreased 30% among women 30 to 69 years old. The decrease in mortality was 61% for ages 30 to 39 years, 53% for ages 40 to 49, 26% for ages 50 to 59, and virtually no change was seen among women 60 years of age and older.

FINLAND (Hakama, 1985; Laara et al, 1987): Population screening began in the early 1960s. Screening usually begins at age 30 and continues to age 55. Women are invited for screening every five years. Seventy to 80% of women invited to screening attend. The number of screening examinations per year in the program increased from about 2,000 in 1963 to about 120,000 in 1980. Substantially more tests are done outside the program than within it. The cervical cancer mortality rate remained essentially constant, with some fluctuations, during the period 1953 to 1965. The mortality decreased 54% from 1963–1967 to 1978–1982 among women 30 to 69 years old. The decrease in mortality was 72% for ages 30 to 39 years, 77% for ages 40 to 49, 60% for ages 50 to 59, and 32% for ages 60 to 69.

ICELAND (Johannesson et al, 1978, 1982; Laara et al, 1987): Of the five Nordic countries, the most intensive screening was done in Iceland. Population screening began in 1964. Women are invited for screening every two to three years. At the start of the program it was limited to women who lived in the area of the capital city and who were 25 to 59 years old. From 1969 onward screening was country-wide and women up to 70 years of age were included. As of 1978, about 85% of women 25 to 59 years old had been screened at least once. Compliance was highest among women 30 to 39 years old: Over 90% of these women had been screened. In 1987 the compliance of women 25 to 69 years old was stated to be 80%. Cervical cancer mortality rates were based on all deaths among diagnosed cases of cervical cancer in order to accommodate changes in accuracy of certification of cause of death. The mortality rate decreased 73% from 1963–1967 to 1975–1979. The decrease in mortality was proportionally greatest among women aged 30 to 39; the rate fell from 7.0 to 0.0 per 100,000 PY. Proportional decreases of 66% or more were seen through age 69.

NORWAY (Hakama, 1982; Laara et al, 1987; Magnus et al, 1987): Norway has had the least population screening of any Scandinavian country. A program in one county began in 1959. Women 25 to 59 years old were invited to participate. These women represented about five percent of the national total in this age group. Originally, the interval between examinations was two years. More recently it has been three to four years. At the first screen, attendance was 76% of women invited. At subsequent screens, 55 to 59% of invited women attended. In contrast to other Nordic countries, cervical cancer mortality in Norway fell during the decade before 1963, although it has been suggested that the increasing rates elsewhere are the result of improvement in the accuracy of reporting. From 1963–1967 to 1978–1982, cervical cancer mortality in Norway fell by eight percent. The decrease is smaller than it was in any other Nordic country during the same period, and it is a substantially smaller decrease than occurred during the preceding decade. For women aged 30 to 49 years, mortality from cervical cancer decreased about 35%. This was the smallest decrease in this age group among the Nordic countries. Cervical cancer mortality either increased or remained essentially constant among Norwegian women in other age groups.

SWEDEN (Hakama, 1982; Laara et al, 1987; Pettersson et al, 1985): Screening programs began in some areas in 1964. Screening was offered nationwide beginning in 1973. Women 30 to 49 years old are invited to be screened every four years. Compliance with the program has been estimated as 70%. In the decade before 1963, cervical cancer mortality in Sweden increased. From 1963–1967 to 1978–1982, the mortality rate decreased 37%. Mortality decreased a little more than 60% among women 30 to 49 years old. There was a 40% decrease in cervical cancer mortality among women 50 to 59 years old, but little change among women 60 years of age or older.

Laara et al (1987) organized the data from the Nordic countries as a before-and-after correlation study (see chapter 5). Substantial decreases in cervical cancer mortality occurred in each of the four countries with broadly-based organized programs (Table 11–1). The largest decrease occurred in Iceland, where screening was most intensive. There was only a small change in rate in Norway, which had little organized screening. Moreover, the largest decreases in mortality occurred in the age groups that were screened most intensively. As shown in the papers cited above, decreases in the incidence of invasive cervical cancer in relation to screening also were observed.

Additional correlation studies of the effectiveness of cervical cancer screening have come from the United States, Canada, and Great Britain.

Cramer (1974) showed a positive correlation between the frequency of the Pap smear and the decline in cervical cancer mortality from 1950–1954 to 1965–1969 in states in the United States (Figure 5–1). In this analysis, no attempt was made to adjust for possible confounding effects of socioeconomic variables.

Miller et al (1976) described an analysis of Canadian data that was based on deaths from cancer of the entire uterus, rather than the cervix, because the proportion of deaths certified specifically as cancer of the cervix changed at different rates among the provinces during the period of the study. Before 1962, there was little screening for cervical cancer in Canada, except in British Columbia. The change in uterine cancer mortality by province from 1950–1952 to 1960–1962 was virtually uncorrelated with the respective provincial screening rate in 1962. The rate of screening increased during the early 1960s. The amount of the decrease in rate from 1960–1962 to 1970–1972 in each province was strongly correlated with the provincial screening rate in 1966. The effects of controlling indicators of socioeconomic status were evaluated in analyses that made use of data by county or census district. The correlation of screening rate with the subsequent decline in mortality continued to be observed with the adjustments that were made. Adjustments for hysterectomies had only small effects on the observed trends (Miller et al, 1981).

The positive correlation of the decrease in uterine cancer mortality with the intensity of screening as reported in 1976 was not seen in data from later periods (eg, change in mortality 1965–1967 to 1975–1977 with respect to screening in 1971; change in mortality 1970–1972 to 1980–1982 with respect to screening in 1976) (Miller et al, 1981; Miller, 1986). However, conditions may not have been appropriate for a before-and-after correlation analysis in the later period. Intensive screening began earlier in the western part of Canada than it did in the east. The first analysis (Miller et al, 1976) reflects the rapid fall in mortality in western Canada in relation to the intensive screening there, compared to the relatively low rates of screening and decreases of mortality in the east. Later, the greatest changes in mortality were seen in the east, where screening was increasing most rapidly. However, the rates of screening continued to be higher in the west than in the east, so that the higher rates of screening were associated with the smaller changes in mortality. Furthermore, the high rates of screening in the west may, to a greater extent than in the east, be the result of repeat screening, which is likely to be less effective than initial screening is (Miller et al, 1981; Miller, 1986). Despite the ambiguous results of the before-and-after analyses, after-only analyses have consistently shown a protective relation between screening frequency and uterine cancer mortality in Canada (Miller, 1986).

Screening frequencies in 14 English Health Regions and Wales for the periods 1967–1973 and 1974–1984 were analyzed in relation to levels of cervical cancer mortality and changes in mortality from earlier to later periods (Murphy et al, 1988). There was an inverse association of the intensity of screening with the mortality rate at a given time (after-only analysis) but little evidence that the change with time in cervical cancer mortality was associated with the intensity of screening (before-and-after analysis). Although negative, the before-and-after analysis is not persuasive evidence against the value of screening. The intensity of screening did not vary much by area in the United Kingdom compared to Canada, the Nordic countries, or the United States. Thus, the correlation of screening with the trend in cervical cancer mortality in the United Kingdom is likely to have been relatively small and difficult to detect.

In addition to these analyses, screening activities in a given area have been related to cervical cancer mortality or incidence in the same area for

Great Britain (MacGregor and Teper, 1978; Parkin et al, 1985), Canada (Kinlen and Doll, 1973), British Columbia (Anderson et al, 1988), Alberta (Starreveld et al, 1981), the Netherlands (Van der Graaf et al, 1988a), East Germany (Ebeling and Nischan, 1986, 1987), the United States (Gardner and Lyon, 1977), Louisville, Kentucky (Christopherson, 1976), Olmstead County, Minnesota (Dickinson, 1972), and Toledo, Ohio (Kim et al, 1978). Some of these findings were considered by the authors to support the value of screening; other findings were considered to be negative or equivocal.

In British Columbia the level of participation in screening has been very high, with 85% of women being screened at least once and nearly half of women over 20 years of age being screened every year. Mortality from cervical cancer fell 73% over a 27-year period (Anderson et al, 1988).

The results from the Netherlands were reported as "negative." Population screening began nearly a decade later in the Netherlands than it did in some other areas, however, so the trend in cervical cancer mortality might not be expected to change much during the 1970s. The data do suggest an increase in the rate of decline in the early 1980s (Van der Graaf et al, 1988a).

Geographic and time trends of cervical cancer mortality (or incidence) are subject to a number of influences in addition to screening. As described in chapter 5, the mortality (or incidence) may be increasing or decreasing as a result of changes in the distribution of causal factors. In addition, diagnostic accuracy has been improving. Until fairly recently, deaths from cervical cancer may have been certified as cancer of the uterus. The fraction of cervical cancer deaths affected may have been so high that the change in diagnostic practices could have created the appearance of increasing mortality from cervical cancer when the trend was actually decreasing (Miller et al, 1976). Furthermore, hysterectomy is a very common operation. Changes in the frequency of hysterectomy may affect trends in cervical cancer incidence or mortality (Lyon and Gardner, 1977; Marrett, 1980; Miller et al, 1981).

Influences such as these may create errors in the assessment of screening. For example, screening might be associated, through a high level of medical care, with better diagnostic accuracy, which may lead to an apparent increase in mortality. Thus, the value of screening might be underestimated. Hysterectomy might be associated with screening, either through a high level of medical care or as a nonspecific result of screening. If so, the value of screening would be overestimated, unless the frequency of hysterectomy is accommodated in the analysis.

The ascertainment and quantification of screening exposure are additional potential sources of error. It may not be possible to distinguish symptomatic from screen-detected cases of invasive cancer. If not, the effect of screening in reducing the incidence of invasive cancer might be underestimated.

In areas where screening programs have been established, the extent of screening has been estimated from program data without taking account of screening done outside the program. The number of examinations done outside the program may be substantially greater than the number done within it. If the amount of screening done outside programs were unrelated to the amount done within them, this would tend to dampen the results of correlation analyses based on screening done within programs. The actual circumstances, however, are complicated. The existence of a program is likely to affect the frequency of screening by other sources, and it is not generally clear what the effect of screening done outside established programs has had on analyses that have been published.

In other areas, screening is available only through routine medical practice. In analyses of data from such areas, the intensity of screening has been measured as the fraction of women screened in a given period, typically a year. Such averages do not distinguish newly-screened from repetitively-screened women. Repeated examinations may make a large contribution to the average screening frequency. Consider a hypothetical screening program that begins in a previously unscreened population. Each year the program screens for the first time 2% of the women in the population. After 12 years 24% of the women will have been screened at least once. If every woman who is screened once then reappears for screening every year, the per capita intensity of screening in the twelfth year also will be 24%. On the other hand, if every woman who is screened once then reappears every third year, the per capita frequency will be only 8%. Because of the generally long duration of dysplasia and carcinoma in situ of the cervix, frequent rescreening may have only a small effect on mortality. If so, failure to distinguish new from repeated screening may weaken observed correlations. The determination of screening frequencies of individuals in correlation studies, however, may require the linking, by name, of many thousands of cytology reports, a task that is likely to be impractical.

Furthermore, per capita averages are not limited to screening examinations; they also include tests done for clinical indications and repeated tests following unsatisfactory ones. As a result, the fraction of screened women and the frequency of screening among screened women are lower than would otherwise be estimated. These errors also lead to underestimation of the value of screening.

The establishment of screening was a gradual process in most areas, often taking 15 to 20 years from the start to the achievement of a high level of coverage. Therefore any reduction in mortality that is brought about also will occur gradually. The slowness of an expected change in mortality adds to the difficulty of distinguishing the effect of screening from other influences. In an experimental screening program its effect can be timed with respect to the dates on which individual subjects are invited to be screened so that the primary determinant of the rate of change in mortality is the effect of early treatment on the progression of the disease. Similarly, information on the times at which subjects are first screened, or first invited to be screened, could be used to sharpen the appearance of any change caused by the program in before-after analyses.

CASE-CONTROL STUDIES

Methods and Results

These studies are summarized in Table 11–2. The descriptions that follow emphasize aspects of the methods that are discussed subsequently.

Clarke and Anderson (1979) reported a study based on cases aged 20 to 69 who were hospitalized with newly diagnosed invasive carcinoma of the cervix. Controls were matched to the cases by age and neighborhood. The analysis ignored Pap smears done as a result of gynecologic symptoms, tests done within the year of diagnosis for cases, and tests done in the corresponding period for controls. Thirty-two percent of cases and 56% of controls had a Pap smear for screening during the five years before the year of diagnosis. The relative risk of invasive cervical cancer was estimated as 3.3 in women who had not, compared to women who had, been screened.

Aristizabal et al (1984) interviewed 204 cases of invasive cervical cancer who were newly-diagnosed and 73 previously diagnosed cases. Two groups of 277 controls each were interviewed. These were selected from "attendants at the health center or clinic in which the case was diagnosed," and from residents of the neighborhoods in which the cases lived. The analysis was based on a history of screening in the period 12 to 72 months before the date of diagnosis of the case. Only 4.3% of cases reported a history of screening, compared to 52.0% of "health center" controls and 31.0% of "neighborhood controls." The relative risk of cervical cancer in screened compared to unscreened women was estimated as 0.042 by use of health center controls and 0.101 by use of neighborhood controls.

La Vecchia et al (1984) described a hospital-based study in which 191 cases and 191 controls were interviewed with respect to their screening

Table 11–2. Summary of Case-control Studies of the Effect of Screening on the Incidence of Invasive Cervical Cancer

Investigators	Location and case intake period	Number of cases	Number of controls	Percent reduction in cervical cancer incidence
Clark and Anderson (1979)	Toronto, 1973–1976	212	1060	70
Aristizabal et al (1984)	Cali, 1977–1981	277	277	90
La Vecchia et al (1984)	Milan, 1981–1983	191	191	74
Berrino et al (1986)	Milan, 1978	121	350	39
Wangsuphachart et al (1987)	Bangkok, 1979–1983	189	1023	28
Celentano et al (1988)	Maryland, 1982–1984	153	153	80
Olesen (1988)	Denmark, 1983	428	428	71
Van der Graaf et al (1988b)	Nijmegen, 1979–1985	36	120	68
Shy et al (1989)	Washington State, 1978–1983	92	178	56

histories. The investigators excluded from the analysis Pap smears that were "made for diagnostic purposes because of bleeding or other symptoms suggestive of cervical neoplasia." A history of screening was reported by 31% of cases and by 64% of controls. Thus, a crude estimate of the relative risk of invasive cervical cancer in screened compared to unscreened women is 0.26. La Vecchia et al also compared screening histories between women with carcinoma in situ and controls. As carcinoma in situ is asymptomatic and is detected only by screening, this comparison is not directly relevant to the question of whether screening reduces cervical cancer morbidity or mortality.

Berrino et al (1986) identified 121 newly diagnosed cases of invasive cervical cancer of which 12 were diagnosed as a result of a positive Pap smear. Screening histories for these cases and 350 controls were obtained from the records of the laboratories that had examined nearly all Pap smears done in Milan. In assessing screening history, Berrino et al ignored Pap smears done within 12 months of the onset of symptoms of cases (an average of four months before diagnosis) and six months of asymptomatic screen-detected cases, and the corresponding periods before July 1, 1978 for the respective controls. Seventeen percent of cases and 25% of controls had had at least one previous screening examination. Thus, a history of screening was associated with a 39% reduction in incidence.

Wangsuphachart et al (1987) reported a hospital-based study. The cases had newly-diagnosed invasive cancer and were at least 15 years old. Cases (n = 189) and controls (n = 1023) were interviewed with respect to Pap smears that were done "more than six months before diagnosis or hospitalization." Data were not included on "smears that led to diagnosis of invasive cervical cancer." At least one Pap smear was reported by 30% of cases and 37% of controls. From the data in Table 4 of the paper, the risk of invasive cervical cancer can be estimated as 0.72 in screened compared to unscreened women.

Ebeling and Nischan (1986, 1987) carried out a survey of trends in screening and in cervical cancer incidence and mortality in Berlin. As part of the survey, the investigators determined the screening histories of women with invasive cervical cancer and of a sample of the female population. A screened woman was defined as one who had at least one Pap test during an interval that varied from 4½ to 5½ years preceding the six-month period before the diagnosis of invasive cervical cancer. Both incidence and mortality were reported to be substantially reduced in screened women. However, some of the information on which the results were based, such as the number and screening histories of the cervical cancer deaths, was not presented.

Celentano et al (1988) identified 153 patients with invasive cervical cancer who had been referred to an oncology department. Cases and controls were matched according to age, race, and neighborhood. Screening histories were obtained by interview. For each matched set, screening through the year before the diagnosis of the case was recorded. There were 28.1% of cases and 7.2% of controls who had never had a Pap test. From these percentages, the risk of invasive cervical cancer can be estimated as 0.20 in screened compared to unscreened women.

Olesen (1988) used a population cancer registry to identify cases of invasive cervical cancer. Controls were selected from the rolls of the respective general practitioners, and the screening histories were obtained from questionnaires completed by the general practitioners. For each case-control pair, information was obtained on "routine" screening examinations done up to the date on which the case was first suspected of having cervical cancer. Of 428 cases, 329 were diagnosed as a result of symptoms or signs other than an abnormal smear. Forty-five percent of the cases and 67% of the controls had been screened more than six months before the respective date on which cervical cancer was first suspected. The relative risk of cervical cancer in screened compared to unscreened women was estimated as 0.29 (0.15–0.56). This estimate was based only on cases that had not been diagnosed as a result of screening, and for whom the most recent test before the diagnosis was done for "routine screening."

Van der Graaf et al (1988b) used a cancer registry to identify cases who had had newly diagnosed invasive cervical cancer, stage Ib or higher, and who were younger than 70 years of age at the time of diagnosis. Of 67 cases identified, 64 were diagnosed clinically and three were detected in a screening program. Controls were selected from population registers. The analysis was based on 36 cases and 120 controls for whom screening histories could be obtained with a mail questionnaire supplemented by personal interview. Forty-seven percent of the cases had been screened at least once, compared to 68 percent of the controls. The estimated relative risk of cervical cancer in screened compared to unscreened women was 0.32 (0.12–0.87, 95% confidence interval).

Shy et al (1989) identified cases through a population-based tumor registry. An attempt was made to restrict the case series to women whose diagnosis followed the occurrence of symptoms. Women diagnosed with microinvasive (stage Ia) or asymptomatic occult (stage Ib-occult) cervical cancer were not eligible. Women with stage Ib or more advanced disease were considered to be eligible unless the tumor registry abstract stated that there had been no symptoms. The case series included two cases with previous stage Ib-occult disease who had had symptomatic recurrences during the intake period. Two potential cases and six potential controls were excluded because they had been treated for carcinoma in situ of the cervix before the study period. Controls were selected by random-digit dialing. The analysis was based on data obtained by interview of 92 cases and 178 controls. "Responses were restricted to events that occurred before the month and year of diagnosis, or before the reference date . . . Papanicolaou smears collected in the follow-up of an abnormal or atypical Papanicolaou smear were excluded, as were Papanicolaou smears obtained at the diagnosis of a cervical cancer." Eighty-five percent of the cases and 93% of the controls had been screened during the 10-year period ending at the reference date. By use of data in Table 2 of the paper, the crude relative risk of cervical cancer in screened compared to unscreened women can be estimated as 0.44.

Methodologic issues

Each of these studies has shown a lower risk of cervical cancer in screened compared to unscreened women. As shown in the original reports, furthermore, most of the associations were not strongly affected by control of potential confounding variables. Nonetheless, there are aspects of the designs of these studies that limit their value.

Most of the studies were based on incident cases of cervical cancer, not advanced metastatic cases or cervical cancer deaths. There are practical reasons for this: The frequencies of these serious outcomes are low, and it is difficult to obtain accurate screening histories of comparable quality for dead cases and live controls. As a result, however, most of the data do not bear directly on the effectiveness of screening in reducing disability or death from cervical cancer. Shy et al (1989) attempted to limit the case series to women with disease diagnosed as a result of symptoms, but in other studies the case series included asymptomatic invasive cancers. The importance of choosing an appropriate outcome event was emphasized in chapter 4. Since asymptomatic invasive cancer is detected by screening, the inclusion of such cases tends to reduce the apparent value of screening (Morrison, 1983). The size of the error depends, among other things, on the frequency of screening, which affects the fraction of the case series that is asymptomatic. The reported fraction of such cases has varied from 4 to 23%.

Patients who develop invasive cancer but who were diagnosed initially in the in situ phase should be included in the case series, but this may not have been done in studies that were based on newly diagnosed invasive disease. Assuming that initial diagnoses of carcinoma in situ are the result of screening, cases that later become invasive represent "failures" of early treatment and their exclusion would artificially inflate the apparent value of screening.

It can be difficult to distinguish a test done for screening from one that is done in the course of diagnosing symptomatic disease. Therefore some investigators have excluded from consideration as screening those tests done in the six months or year preceding the diagnosis (and the equivalent period for controls). Diagnostic examinations erroneously considered to be screening tend to reduce the apparent value of screening, since a higher proportion of cases than of controls would be expected to have had tests as a result of symptoms. However, the exclusion of all tests within some period ending at diagnosis also tends to reduce the apparent value of screening, if any, because some of the screening examinations that lead to early treatment would be ignored. The only test that can be beneficial is a confirmed positive.

In analyses of incidence risk between screened and unscreened persons, there is no intermediate disease event that predicts the occurrence of invasive cervical cancer and that would preclude having at least one screening examination. Therefore, comparisons of ever-screened v unscreened persons are not affected by healthy-screenee bias (see chapter 5). Continued screening, however, depends on negative results in previous screens. Data on the relation of frequency of screening to risk of cervical cancer has been presented for most of the case-control studies. With one exception (Berrino et al, 1986), however, these analyses did not accommodate the potential for healthy-screenee bias, so the results may tend to overestimate the benefit of frequent screening. Consequently, the information is of uncertain value in formulating screening policy.

Some studies have restricted the consideration of screening tests to those done during a period typically five or ten years long that ends at or shortly before the time of diagnosis. Presumably this restriction is intended to increase the accuracy of screening histories. This procedure, however, may create healthy-screenee bias. Screening behavior before the period may predict both the screening behavior during the period and the subsequent risk of the outcome. Persons who have several negative screens before the start of the exposure "window" are more likely than others to seek screening again during the window, and persons with several previous negative screens are relatively unlikely to develop symptomatic invasive disease. The size of an error introduced by use of an exposure window is unknown. Any error, however, is likely to decrease in importance as the window occupies an increasingly large portion of the period of life in which screening is relevant.

Some studies have presented data on the change in the protective effect of screening with time after the most recent examination. Such analyses should be designed so that time since the most recent exam is not associated with risk except through a protective effect. In case-control studies, events are usually timed with respect to diagnosis, not exposure. Other things being equal, a case or control who has been screened frequently is more likely to have had a recent examination than is a subject who has been screened infrequently. Since screening frequency is a determinant of time since examination, such analyses also may be affected by healthy-screenee bias.

In several of the studies, screening histories could not be obtained from a high proportion of cases. In some instances a high proportion of those identified had died by the time the study was done. It is not always clear what fraction of controls was interviewed. In some studies the proportion of controls not interviewed was quite high. Some investigators were able to compare screening histories obtained by interview with histories derived from records, or to compare recorded histories between interview respondents and nonrespondents (Aristizabal et al, 1984; Clarke and Anderson, 1979; Van der Graaf et al, 1988; Wangsuphachart et al, 1987). The histories obtained by interview were found to be reasonably accurate. The discrepancies found have been reasonably small, and the types of errors that were made indicate that the observed effect of screening tends to be less than the true effect (Clarke and Anderson, 1979; Van der Graaf et al, 1988).

AN INDIRECT APPROACH

The time trend of the incidence rate of symptomatic disease following a negative screening examination depends on the distribution of the duration of preclinical disease. This trend may be estimated by either the follow-up or case-control method (Walter and Day, 1983; Brookmeyer et al, 1986). Assuming that the early treatment of positive cases prevents their progression to symptomatic disease, however, all symptomatic disease in screened persons would occur among those who test negative. The time trend of symptomatic disease following a negative screening examination suggests the value of various screening intervals at keeping the occurrence of symptomatic disease at acceptably low levels.

It is important to emphasize that this approach to the evaluation of screening is indirect. The trend of incidence following a negative screening examination does not, by itself, indicate the efficacy of early treatment. Use of a sensitive test will lead to a low rate of symptomatic disease shortly after a negative examination even if early treatment is not beneficial.

A combined analysis of the trend in the incidence of invasive cervical cancer following a negative screen in several geographic areas was reported by an IARC Working Group (1986). Since the analysis focused on women who had had at least two negative examinations, the trend is unlikely to have been influenced much by incident cases that had been false negatives. The relative incidence was very low in the first few years after screening, rising to the expected value after about ten years. The authors used the data to estimate the cumulative reduction in incidence in women 20 to 64 years of age that would be achieved by various screening policies (Table 11–3). Yearly screening appears only slightly better than screening every three years. Screening every five years appears somewhat less effective than screening every three years. The results suggest a response curve like that in Figure 8–1. There would be little additional benefit from starting to screen at age 20 compared with age 25 because of the low incidence of the disease in the young (IARC Working Group, 1986). There would be some gain from starting to screen at age 25 instead of age 35.

The data in Table 11–3 imply the effect of screening at various intervals on cervical cancer mortality. The *relative* effect of screening on mortality would be similar to the relative effect of screening on incidence provided that the time after screening at which a case is detected and treated is not strongly related to its subsequent rate of progression. On the other hand, screening is likely to have a stronger *arithmetic* effect on the incidence of invasive cancer than it does on mortality from the disease since the mortality rate from cancer of the cervix is less than the incidence rate even in the absence of screening. Thus, not every screen-detected case benefits from early treatment; some cases might be cured by treatment at the time that symptoms develop because metastasis has not yet occurred.

Table 11-3. Estimated Percentage Reduction in Cumulative Incidence of Invasive Cervical Cancer in Women Aged 20 to 64 Years Achieved by Various Screening Policies

Policy		
Interval of screening in years	Ages of screening	Percent reduction in cumulative incidence
1	20–64	93
3	20–64	91
5	20–64	84
3	25–64	90
3	35–64	78
5	25–64	82
5	35–64	70

Source: Adapted from IARC Working Group (1986).

As the authors indicated, the data shown imply more rapid progression of the disease than may occur. Symptomatic cases of invasive cancer were not separated from asymptomatic cases detected by screening. Such cases are detected earlier than they would be otherwise, elevating the incidence rate following a negative screening test. In some of the areas, such cases were a high proportion of the total. Furthermore, early treatment may benefit asymptomatic cases of invasive cancer detected by screening. Thus, somewhat less frequent screening than is implied by their results might be appropriate. On the other hand, the data were derived from women who were screened. The relation of the rate of progression of cervical cancer to willingness to be screened is not known.

CONCLUSIONS

Cytologic screening for cervical cancer is an effective measure for reducing morbidity and mortality from cervical cancer. This conclusion is supported by most of the geographic correlation and time trend analyses and all of the case-control studies that are summarized. Some before-and-after correlation analyses have been negative, but this is not strong contradictory evidence, as explained above.

All the evidence on the effectiveness of screening for cervical cancer is nonexperimental. It is possible that the risk of cervical cancer differs systematically between screened and unscreened women for reasons other than screening. Given the consistency of the evidence assembled by different methods and based on diverse sources, and the results of controlling known potential confounding variables, it is unlikely that confounding variables are responsible for most of the apparent value of screening.

Screening a high fraction of women is associated with a reduction in cervical cancer mortality of roughly two thirds to three fourths. Proportionally this is the most effective known type of screening for a chronic disease of adults. Although even higher reductions may be achievable, it is unrealistic to expect that cervical cancer mortality can be eliminated entirely by screening. Inevitably, some women will not be screened at all, or will not reappear at prescribed intervals; some cases of the disease will develop too fast to be detected by screening at a frequency that is practical; some screened cases will be erroneously reported as negative; and some screen-detected cases will not be managed correctly (Chamberlain, 1986).

In many areas cervical cancer mortality is low as a result of screening that has been available for 20 years or more. New screening programs in such areas cannot have a large arithmetic effect.

Screening is effective for women 30 to 69 years old. Little direct information is available on the value of screening outside this range. In a number of studies, the age distributions of screenees has not been specified.

Useful data are not available on the relative efficacy of screening according to age. If it is roughly constant, the ages at which screening should be done depend on the incidence of early cervical cancer and the rate at which it would progress past the point at which early detection and treatment is effective. Cervical cancer incidence and mortality are very low in young women. There is probably not much value in starting to screen before age 25. Cervical dysplasia and carcinoma in situ progress relatively slowly. Screening that begins at about age 25 should bring about a large reduction in the increasing incidence and mortality in the 30s, 40s, and later.

The upper age limit for screening depends, again, on the incidence of early cancer, on the interval from early detection to the time at which the benefit of reduced morbidity or mortality is realized, and on the rates of competing causes of death. The longer the interval, and the higher the rates, the earlier screening should be ended.

Screening every two to three years appears to be more effective than less frequent screening. None of the evidence suggests that annual screening is much more effective than is screening every two to three years. Given the many sources of systematic and random variability that influence the data, it is difficult to be confident of the amount of reduction in mortality gained by screening every two to three years v less often. It is not possible to distinguish the value of screening every four years v every five years.

A high proportion of false negatives has been taken as a reason for yearly as opposed to less frequent screening. The frequency of false negatives may be estimated by comparing the incidence of invasive disease following one v two or more negative tests. In some areas the frequency of false negatives may be as high as 40% (IARC Working Group, 1986). Nonetheless, the generally long duration of dysplasia or carcinoma in situ insures that nearly all false negatives will be detected subsequently while still noninvasive by screening at two- or three-year intervals. Furthermore, a policy of annual screening unnecessarily increases both false positives and costs.

Other things being equal, the efficiency of screening at a given frequency—the reduction in morbidity and mortality in relation to the medical and economic costs—can be improved by the restriction of screening to high risk groups (see chapter 7). Such restriction involves a judgment as to whether the gain in efficiency outweighs the loss of some of the benefit of screening to the total population. There would be virtually no loss in excluding from screening, if practical, women who have not had sexual intercourse. Restriction of screening to groups defined by marital status or social class may lead to unacceptably large losses in benefit to the total population (Hakama, 1979, 1986). Age is a useful indicator of high risk. As indicated above, there is little point in screening very young women.

Indicators of risk might also be viewed as guides to the frequency of rescreening. A recommendation for frequent rescreening of high-risk groups would be appropriate, for example, if more frequent screening were necessary to achieve a given proportional level of disease control in high-risk as compared to low-risk groups. This might be the case if the rate of progression of preclinical cervical cancer were correlated with its incidence. Useful evidence on this question, however, is not available (Hakama, 1986).

References

Albert A, Gertman PM, Louis TA: Screening for the early detection of cancer: I. The temporal natural history of a progressive disease state. *Math Biosci* 1978a; 40:1–59.

Albert A, Gertman PM, Louis TA, Liu S-I: Screening for the early detection of cancer: II. The impact of screening on the natural history of the disease. *Math Biosci* 1978b; 40:61–109.

Alexander HR, Candela FC, Dershaw DD, Kinne DW: Needle-localized mammographic lesions. Results and evolving treatment strategy. *Arch Surg* 1990; 125:1441–1444.

American Cancer Society: Guidelines for the cancer-related check-up: recommendations and rationale. *Ca–A Cancer Journal for Clinicians* 1980; 30:194–240.

American Cancer Society's National Task Force on Breast Cancer Control, 1982: Mammography 1982: a statement of the American Cancer Society. *Ca–A Cancer Journal for Clinicians* 1982; 32:226–230.

Anderson GH, Boyes DA, Benedet JL, et al: Organisation and results of the cervical cytology screening programme in British Columbia, 1955–85. *Br Med J* 1988; 296:975–978.

Anderson TJ, Alexander F, Chetty U, et al: Comparative pathology of prevalent and incident cancers detected by breast screening. *Lancet* 1986; i:519–523.

Andersson I, Aspergren K, Janzon L, et al: Mammographic screening and mortality from breast cancer: the Malmo mammographic screening trial. *Br Med J* 1988; 297:943–948.

Aristizabal N, Cuello C, Correa P, et al: The impact of vaginal cytology on cervical cancer risks in Cali, Columbia. *Int J Cancer* 1984; 34:5–9.

Armitage P, Fox W, Rose GA, Tinker CM: The variability of measurements of causal blood pressure: II. Survey experience. *Clin Sci* 1966; 30:337–344.

Aron JL, Prorok PC: Analysis of the age mortality effect in a breast cancer screening study. *Int J Epidemiol* 1986; 15:36–43.

Association for the Prevention and Relief of Heart Disease. *First Report.* New York, 1921.

Baines CJ: Breast self-examination. *Cancer* 1989; 64 (suppl):2661–2663.

Baines CJ: Breast self-examination: the known and the unknown, in Day NE, Miller AB (eds): *Screening for Breast Cancer.* Toronto, Huber, 1988, pp 85–91.

Baker LH: Breast cancer detection demonstration project: five-year summary report. *Ca–A Cancer Journal for Clinicians* 1982; 32:194–225.

Beahrs OH, Shapiro S, Smart C: Report of the working group to review the National Cancer Institute—American Cancer Society Breast Cancer Detection Demonstration Projects. *JNCI* 1979; 62:640–709.

Berrino F, Gatta G, D'Alto M, Crosignani P: Efficacy of screening in preventing invasive cervical cancer: a case-control study in Milan, Italy, in Hakama M, Miller AB, Day NE (eds): *Screening for Cancer of the Uterine Cervix.* Lyon, International Agency for Research on Cancer, 1986, pp 111–123.

Berwick M, Roush G, Thompson WD: Evaluating the efficacy of skin self-exam and other surveillance measures in persons at various levels of risk for cutaneous malignant melanoma: an ongoing case-control study, in Anderson PN, Engstrom PF, Mortenson LE (eds): *Advances in Cancer Control: Innovations and Research.* New York, Alan R. Liss, 1985, pp 297–305.

Bishop YMM, Fienberg SE, Holland PW: *Discrete Multivariate Analysis: Theory and Practice.* Cambridge, Mass, MIT Press, 1975.

Blalock HM Jr: *Causal Inferences in Nonexperimental Research.* Chapel Hill, The University of North Carolina Press, 1964.

Bodian D, Horstmann DM: Polioviruses, in Horsfall FL, Tamm I (eds): *Viral and Rickettsial Infections of Man,* ed 4. Philadelphia, Lippincott, 1965, pp 430–473.

Boice JD Jr, Preston D, Davis FG, Monson RR: Frequent chest x-ray fluoroscopy and breast cancer incidence among tuberculosis patients in Massachusetts. *Radiat Res* 1991; 125:214–222.

Boyes DA, Morrison B, Knox EG, et al: A cohort study of cervical cancer screening in British Columbia. *Clin Invest Med* 1982; 5:1–29.

Breslow L, Wilner D, Agran L, et al: *A History of Cancer Control in the United States, 1946–1971. Book One: A History of Scientific and Technical Advances in Cancer Control.* US Dept of Health, Education, and Welfare, National Cancer Institute, 1979, pp 201–218.

Breslow L, Thomas LB, Upton AC: Final reports. The NCI ad hoc working groups on mammography in screening for breast cancer and a summary report of their joint findings and recommendations. *JNCI* 1977; 59:468–541.

Breslow NE, Day NE: *Statistical Methods in Cancer Research: Volume 1—The Analysis of Case-Control Studies.* Lyon, International Agency for Research on Cancer, 1980.

Breslow NE, Day NE: *Statistical Methods in Cancer Research: Volume 2—The Design and Analysis of Cohort Studies.* Lyon, International Agency for Research on Cancer, 1987.

Brett GZ: The value of lung cancer detection by six-monthly chest radiographs. *Thorax* 1968; 23:414–420.

Brisson J, Merletti F, Sadowsky NL, et al: Mammographic features of the breast and breast cancer risk. *Am J Epidemiol* 1982a; 115:428–437.

Brisson J, Morrison AS, Khalid N: Mammographic parenchymal features and breast cancer in the Breast Cancer Detection Demonstration Project. *J Natl Cancer Inst* 1988; 80:1534–1540.

Brisson J, Morrison AS, Kopans DB, et al: Height and weight, mammographic features of breast tissue, and breast cancer risk. *Am J Epidemiol* 1984; 119:371–381.

Brisson J, Sadowsky NL, Twaddle JA, et al: The relation of mammographic features of the breast to breast cancer risk factors. *Am J Epidemiol* 1982b; 115:438–43.

British Medical Journal: Prognosis after myocardial infarction. *Br Med J* 1979; 2:1311–1312.

Brookmeyer R, Day NE, Moss S: Case-control studies for estimation of the natural history of preclinical disease from screening data. *Stat Med* 1986; 5:127–138.

Cartwright RA, Gadian T, Garland JB, et al: The influence of malignant cell cytology screening on the survival of industrial bladder cancer cases. *J Epidemiol Comm Health* 1981; 35:35–38.

Celentano DD, Klassen AC, Weisman CS, Rosenshein NB: Cervical cancer screening practices among older women: results from the Maryland cervical cancer case-control study. *J Clin Epidemiol* 1988; 41:531–541.

Chamberlain J: Breast self-examination. Paper presented at the UICC Multidisciplinary Project on Breast Cancer. Meeting on Screening, Detection, and Diagnosis, Leeds Castle, England, 1982.

Chamberlain J: Reasons that some screening programs fail to control cervical cancer, in Hakama M, Miller AB, Day NE (eds): *Screening for Cancer of the Uterine Cervix*. Lyon, International Agency for Research on Cancer, 1986, pp 161–168.

Chamberlain J, Clifford RE, Nathan BE, et al: Repeated screening for breast cancer. *J Epidemiol Comm Health* 1984; 38:54–57.

Chiang CL: A stochastic study of the life table and its applications: III. The follow-up study with the consideration of competing risks. *Biometrics* 1961; 17:57–78.

Chen JS, Prorok P: Lead time estimation in a controlled screening program. *Am J Epidemiol* 1983; 118:740–751.

Christopherson WM, Lundin FE, Mendez WM, Parker JE: Cervical cancer control. A study of morbidity and mortality trends over a twenty-one year period. *Cancer* 1976; 35:1357–1366.

Clark RL, Copeland MM, Egan RL, et al: Reproducibility of the technique of mammography (Egan) for cancer of the breast. *Amer J Surg* 1965; 109:127–133.

Clarke EA, Anderson TW: Does screening by "Pap" smears help prevent cervical cancer? *Lancet* 1979; 2:1–4.

Cole P: A population-based study of bladder cancer, in Doll R, Vodopija I (eds): *Host Environmental Interactions in the Etiology of Cancer in Man—Implementations in Research*. Lyon, International Agency for Research on Cancer, 1973, pp 83–87.

Cole P, Morrison AS: Basic issues in population screening for cancer. *JNCI* 1980; 64:1263–1272.

Collette HJA, Day NE, Rombach JJ, De Waard F: Evaluation of screening for breast cancer in a non-randomized study (the DOM project) by means of a case control study. *Lancet* 1984; i:1224–1226.

Commission on Chronic Illness: *Chronic Illness in the United States: Prevention of Chronic Illness*. Cambridge, Mass, Harvard University Press, 1957; 47:601–607.

Committee of Principal Investigators: A co-operative trial in the primary prevention of ischaemic heart disease using clofibrate. *Br Heart J* 1978; 40:1069–1118.

Committee of Principal Investigators: WHO cooperative trial on primary prevention of ischaemic heart disease with clofibrate to lower serum cholesterol: final mortality follow-up. *Lancet* 1984; ii:600–604.

Cornfield J: The estimation of the probability of developing a disease in the presence of competing risks. *Amer J Pub Health* 1957; 47:601–607.

The Coronary Drug Project Research Group: Influences of adherence to treatment and response of cholesterol on mortality in the Coronary Drug Project. *N Engl J Med* 1980; 303:1038–1041.

Cramer DW: The role of cervical cytology in the declining morbidity and mortality of cervical cancer. *Cancer* 1974; 34:2018–2027.

Cuckle HS, Wald NJ, Lindenbaum RH: Maternal serum alpha-fetoprotein measurement: a screening test for Down syndrome. *Lancet* 1984; i:926–929.

Cuckle HS, Wald NJ: Principles of screening, in Wald NJ (ed): *Antenatal and Neonatal Screening*. Oxford, Oxford University Press, 1984, pp 1–22.

Cuckle HS, Wald NJ, Cuckle PM: Prenatal screening and diagnosis of neural tube defects in England and Wales in 1985. *Prenatal Diagnosis* 1989; 9:393–400.

Cutler SJ, Axtell LM, Schottenfeld D: Adjustment of long-term survival rates for deaths due to intercurrent disease. *J Chron Dis* 1969; 22:485–491.

Dales LG, Friedman GD, Collen MF: Evaluating periodic multiphasic health checkups: a controlled trial. *J Chron Dis* 1979; 32:385–404.

Day NE: Estimating the sensitivity of a screening test. *J Epidemiol Comm Health* 1985; 39:364–366.

Dickinson L, Mussey ME, Soule EH, Kurland LT: Evaluation of the effectiveness of cytologic screening for cervical cancer: I. Incidence and mortality trends in relation to screening. *Mayo Clinic Proc* 1972; 47:534–544.

Doll R, Peto R: The causes of cancer. *JNCI* 1981; 66:1191–1308.

Dubin N: Benefits of screening for breast cancer: Application of a probabilistic model to a breast cancer detection project. *J Chron Dis* 1979; 32:145–151.

Dunn JE Jr: The relationship between carcinoma in situ and invasive cervical carcinoma. *Cancer* 1953; 6:873–886.

Ebeling K, Nischan P: Assessing the effectiveness of a cervical cancer screening program in the German Democratic Republic. *Int J Technology Assessment in Health Care* 1987; 3:137–147.

Ebeling K, Nischan P: Organization and results of cervical cancer screening in the German Democratic Republic, in Hakama M, Miller AB, Day NE (eds): *Screening for Cancer of the Uterine Cervix*. Lyon, International Agency for Research on Cancer, 1986, pp 251–266.

Ebeling K, Nischan P: Screening for lung cancer—results from a case-control study. *Int J Cancer* 1987; 40:141–144.

Eddy DM: *Screening for Cancer: Theory, Analysis and Design*. Englewood Cliffs, Prentice-Hall, 1980.

Eddy DM, Shwartz M: Mathematical models in screening, in Schottenfeld D, Fraumeni JF Jr (eds): *Cancer Epidemiology and Prevention*. Philadelphia, Saunders, 1982, pp 1075–1090.

Ederer F, Axtell LM, Cutler SJ: The relative survival rate: a statistical methodology. *Natl Cancer Inst Monogr* 1961; 6:101–121.

Egan RL: Mammography as an aid to diagnosis of breast carcinoma. *JAMA* 1962; 182:839–843.

Elandt-Johnson RC: Definitions of rates: some remarks on their use and misuse. *Am J Epidemiol* 1975; 102:267–271.

Enterline PE: Pitfalls in epidemiological research: an examination of the asbestos literature. *J Occ Med* 1976; 18:150–156.

Fagerberg CJG, Tabar L: The results of periodic one-view mammography screening in a randomized, controlled trial in Sweden. Part 1: Background, organization, screening program, tumor findings, in Day NE, Miller AB (eds): *Screening for Breast Cancer.* Toronto, Hans Huber, 1988, pp 33–38.

Farrow GM: Pathologist's role in bladder cancer. *Semin Oncol* 1979; 6:198–206.

Feinleib M, Zelen M: Some pitfalls in the evaluation of screening programs. *Arch Environ Health* 1969; 19:412–415.

Ferrer HP: *Screening for Health: Theory and Practice.* London, Butterworths, 1968.

Flanders WD, Longini IM Jr: Estimating benefits of screening from observational cohort studies. *Stat Med* 1990; 9:969–980.

Flehinger BJ, Herbert E, Winawer SJ, Miller DG: Screening for colorectal cancer with fecal occult blood test and sigmoidoscopy: preliminary report of the colon project of Memorial Sloan-Kettering Cancer Center and PMI-Strang Clinic, in Chamberlain J, Miller AB (eds): *Screening for Gastrointestinal Cancer.* Toronto, Hans Huber, 1988, pp 9–16.

Fontana RS: Screening for lung cancer, in Miller AB (ed): *Screening for Cancer.* Orlando, FL, Academic Press, 1985, pp 377–395.

Foster RS Jr, Lang SP, Costanza MD, et al: Breast self-examination practices and breast-cancer stage. *N Engl J Med* 1978; 299:265–270.

Fox AJ, Collier PF: Low mortality rates in industrial cohort studies due to selection for work and survival in the industry. *Br J Prev Soc Med* 1976; 30:225–230.

Francis T, Korns RF, Voight RB, et al: An evaluation of the 1954 poliomyelitis vaccine trial: summary report. *Am J Public Health* 1955; 45:1–63.

Frankenburg WK: Criteria in screening test selection, in Frankenburg WK, Camp BW (eds): *Pediatric Screening Tests.* Springfield, Il, Charles C Thomas, 1975, pp 23–37.

Fraser GE: *Preventive Cardiology.* New York, Oxford University Press, 1986.

Fraumeni JF Jr, Blot WJ: Lung and pleura, in Schottenfeld D, Fraumeni JF Jr (eds): *Cancer Epidemiology and Prevention.* Philadelphia, Saunders, 1982, pp 564–582.

Freeman J, Hutchison GB: Prevalence, incidence and duration. *Am J Epidemiol* 1980; 112:707–723.

Frick MH, Elo O, Haapa K, et al: Helsinki heart study: primary-prevention trial with gemfibrozil in middle-aged men with dyslipidemia. *N Engl J Med* 1987; 317:1237–1245.

Friedman GD, Collen MF, Fireman BH: Multiphasic health checkup evaluation: a 16-year follow up. *J Chron Dis* 1986; 39:453–463.

Fries ED: Should mild hypertension be treated? *N Engl J Med* 1982; 307:306–309.

Frisell J, Eklund G, Hellstrom L, et al: Randomized study of mammography screening—preliminarily report on mortality in the Stockholm trial. *Breast Cancer Res Treat* 1991; 18:49–56.

Gail M: Measuring the benefit of reduced exposure to carcinogens. *J Chron Dis* 1975; 28:135–147.

Gardner JW, Lyon JL: Efficacy of cervical cytologic screening in the control of cervical cancer. *Prev Med* 1977; 6:487–499.

Gentry WD: Psychosocial concerns and benefits in cardiac rehabilitation, in Pollock ML, Schmidt DH (eds): *Heart Disease and Rehabilitation.* Boston, Houghton-Mifflin, 1979, pp 690–700.

Gershon-Cohen J, Hermel MB, Berger SM: Detection of breast cancer by periodic x-ray examination. *JAMA* 1961; 176:1114–1116.

Gilbertsen VA, McHugh R, Schuman L, et al: The early detection of colorectal cancers: a preliminary report of the results of the occult blood study. *Cancer* 1980; 45:2899–2901.

Gilbertsen VA, Nelms JM: The prevention of invasive cancer of the rectum. *Cancer* 1978; 41:1137–1139.

Greenland S: The effect of misclassification in the presence of covariates. *Am J Epidemiol* 1980; 112:564–569.

Greenland S, Thomas DC: On the need for the rare disease assumption in case-control studies. *Am J Epidemiol* 1982; 116:547–553.

Greenough RB, Ewing J, Wainwright JM: *Essential Facts About Cancer: A Handbook for the Medical Profession.* New York, American Society for the Control of Cancer, 1924, pp 27–31.

Haggard HH: *Devils, Drugs, and Doctors.* New York, Harper, 1929, pp 263–264.

Hakama M: Effect of population screening for carcinoma of the uterine cervix in Finland. *Maturitas* 1985; 7:3–10.

Hakama M: Trends in the incidence of cervical cancer in the Nordic countries, in Magnus K (ed): *Trends in Cancer Incidence.* Washington, Hemisphere Publishing Corporation, 1982, pp 279–292.

Hakama M, Pakkala E, Saastamoinen P: Selective screening: theory and practice based on high-risk groups of cervical cancer. *J Epidemiol Comm Health* 1979; 33:257–261.

Helgeland A: Treatment of mild hypertension: a five year controlled drug trial. *Am J Med* 1980; 69:725–732.

Hennekens CH, Buring JE: *Epidemiology in Medicine.* Boston, Little Brown & Co, 1987.

Hill GB, Burns PE, Koch M, et al: Trends in the incidence of cancer of the female breast and reproductive tract in Alberta, 1953 to 1977. *Prev Med* 1983; 12:296–303.

Hjermann I, Velve Byre K, Holme I, Leren P: Effect of diet and smoking intervention on the incidence of coronary heart disease. *Lancet* 1981, ii:1303–1310.

Hoover R, Mason TJ, McKay FW, et al: Geographic patterns of cancer mortality in the United States, in Fraumeni JF Jr (ed): *Persons at High Risk of Cancer.* New York, Academic Press, 1975, pp 343–360.

Howe GR, Burch JD, Miller AB, et al: Tobacco use, occupation, coffee, various nutrients, and bladder cancer. *JNCI* 1980; 64:701–713.

Hutchison GB: Evaluation of preventive services. *J Chron Dis* 1960; 11:497–508.

Hutchison GB: Experimental trial and program review, in Clark DW, MacMahon B (eds): *Preventive and Community Medicine,* ed 2. Boston, Little Brown & Co, 1981, pp 81–95.

Hutchison GB, Shapiro S: Lead time gained by diagnostic screening for breast cancer. *JNCI* 1968; 41:665–681.

Hypertension Detection and Follow-up Program Cooperative Group: Five-year findings of the Hypertension Detection and Follow-up Program: I. reduction in mortality of persons with high blood pressure, including mild hypertension. *JAMA* 1979; 242:2562–2571.

International Agency for Research on Cancer: *Evaluation of the Carcinogenic Risk of Chemicals to Humans: Tobacco Smoking*, vol 38. Lyon, International Agency for Research on Cancer, 1986.

International Agency for Research on Cancer Working Group on Evaluation of Cervical Cancer Screening Programmes: Screening for squamous cervical cancer: duration of low risk after negative results of cervical cytology and its implication for screening policies. *Br Med J* 1986; 293:659–664.

Johannesson G, Geirsson G, Day N: The effect of mass screening in Iceland, 1965–1974, on the incidence and mortality of cervical cancer. *Int J Cancer* 1978; 21:418–425.

Johannesson G, Geirsson G, Day N, Tulinius H: Screening for cancer of the uterine cervix in Iceland 1965–1978. *Acta Obstet Gynecol Scand* 1982; 61:199–203.

Joint National Committee on Detection, Evaluation, and Treatment of High Blood Pressure: The 1984 report of the Joint National Committee on Detection, Evaluation, and Treatment of High Blood Pressure. *Arch Intern Med* 1984; 144:1045–1057.

Kelsey JL: A review of the epidemiology of human breast cancer. *Epidemiol Rev* 1979; 1:74–109.

Kelsey JL, Gammon MD: Update: epidemiology of breast cancer. *Epidemiol Rev* 1990; 12:228–240.

Kim K, Rigel RD, Patrick JR, et al: The changing trends of uterine cancer and cytology. A study of morbidity and mortality trends over a twenty year period. *Cancer* 1978; 42:2439–2449.

Kinlen LJ, Doll R: Trends in mortality from cancer of the uterus in Canada and in England and Wales. *Br J Prev Soc Med* 1973; 27:146–149.

Kleinbaum DG, Kupper LL, Morgenstern H: *Epidemiologic Research: Principles and Quantative Methods.* Belmont, Ca, Lifetime Learning Publications, 1982.

Kopans DB, Meyer JE, Sadowsky N: Breast imaging. *N Engl J Med* 1984; 310:960–967.

Koroltchouk V, Stanley K, Stjernsward J: The control of breast cancer. A World Health Organization perspective. *Cancer* 1990; 65:2803–2810.

Kronborg O, Fenger C, Olsen J, et al: Repeated screening for colorectal cancer with fecal occult blood test. *Scand J Gastroenterol* 1989; 24:599–606.

Kuller LH: Natural history of coronary heart disease, in Pollock ML, Schmidt DH (eds): *Heart Disease and Rehabilitation.* Boston, Houghton-Mifflin, 1979, pp 32–56.

La Vecchia C, Decarli A, Gentile A, et al: "Pap" smear and the risk of cervical neoplasia: quantitative estimates from a case-control study. *Lancet* 1984; ii:779–782.

Laara E, Day N, Hakama M: Trends in mortality from cervical cancer in the Nordic countries: association with organised screening programmes. *Lancet* 1987; i:1247–1249.

Laskey PW, Meigs JW, Flannery JT: Uterine cervical carcinoma in Connecticut, 1935–1973: evidence for two classes of invasive disease. *JNCI* 1976; 57:1037–1043.

Lilienfeld AM, Barnes JM, Barnes RB, et al: An evaluation of thermography in the detection of breast cancer: A cooperative pilot study. *Cancer* 1969; 24:1206–1211.

Lipid Research Clinics Program: The Lipid Research Clinics coronary primary prevention trial results: I. Reduction in incidence of coronary heart disease. *JAMA* 1984; 251:351–364.

Locker AP, Caseldine J, Mitchell AK, et al: Results from a seven-year programme of breast self-examination in 89,010 women. *Br J Cancer* 1989; 60:401–405.

Lundgren B: Efficiency of single-view mammography: rate of interval cases. *JNCI* 1979; 62:799–803.

Lynge E: Regional trends in incidence of cervical cancer in Denmark in relation to local smear-taking activity. *Int J Cancer* 1983; 12:405–413.

Lyon JL, Gardner JW: The rising frequency of hysterectomy: its effect on uterine cancer rates. *Am J Epidemiol* 1977; 105:439–443.

Macgregor JE, Teper S: Mortality from carcinoma of the cervix uteri in Britain. *Lancet* 1978; ii:774–776.

Magnus K, Langmark F, Andersen A: Mass screening for cervical cancer in Ostfold County. *Int J Cancer* 1987; 39:311–316.

Management Committee: The Australian therapeutic trial in mild hypertension. *Lancet* 1980; i:1261–1267.

Marrett LD: Estimates of the true population at risk of uterine disease and an application to incidence data for cancer of the uterine corpus in Connecticut. *Amer J Epidemiol* 1980; 111:373–378.

McClatchey MW, Calonge N, Furmanski P, et al: Results of a community-based breast cancer screening program, in Anderson PN, Engstrom PF, Mortenson LE (eds): *Advances in Cancer Control: Innovations and Research.* New York, Alan R. Liss, 1989, pp 89–101.

Medical Research Council Working Party: MRC trial of treatment of mild hypertension: principal results. *Br Med J* 1985; 291:97–104.

Melamed MR, Flehinger BJ, Zaman MB: Impact of early detection on the clinical course of lung cancer. *Surg Clin N Am* 1987; 67:909–924.

Metropolitan Life Insurance Company: The value of periodic medical examinations. *Stat Bull* 1921; 2:1–2.

Miettinen OS: Estimability and estimation in case-referent studies. *Am J Epidemiol* 1976; 103:226–235.

Miller AB (ed): *Screening in Cancer.* Geneva, International Union Against Cancer, 1978.

Miller AB: Evaluation of the impact of screening for cancer of the cervix, in Hakama M, Miller AB, Day NE (eds): *Screening for Cancer of the Uterine Cervix,* IARC Scientific Publications No. 76. Lyon, International Agency for Research on Cancer, 1986, pp 149–160.

Miller AB, Howe GR, Wall C: The national study of breast cancer screening: protocol for a Canadian randomized controlled trial of screening for breast cancer in women. *Invest Med* 1981a; 4:227–258.

Miller AB, Lindsay JP, Hill GB: Mortality from cancer of the uterus in Canada and its relationship to screening for cancer of the cervix. *Int J Cancer* 1976; 17:602–612.

Miller AB, Visentin T, Howe GR: The effect of hysterectomies and screening on mortality from cancer of the uterus in Canada. *Int J Cancer* 1981b; 27:651–657.

Minutes: UICC Multidisciplinary Project on Breast Cancer. Meeting on Screening, Detection, and Diagnosis, Leeds Castle, England, 1982, p 12.

Monson RR: *Occupational Epidemiology.* Boca Raton, Fl, CRC Press, 1980.

Morgenstern H, Kleinbaum DG, Kupper LL: Measures of disease incidence used in epidemiologic research. *Int J Epidemiol* 1980; 9:97–104.

Morrison AS: Sequential pathogenic components of rates. *Am J Epidemiol* 1979a; 109:709–718.

Morrison AS: The public health value of using epidemiologic information to identify high risk groups for bladder cancer screening. *Semin Oncol* 1979b; 6:184–188.

Morrison AS: Case definition in case-control studies of the efficacy of screening. *Am J Epidemiol* 1982a; 115:6–8.

Morrison AS: The effects of early treatment, lead time, and length bias on the mortality experienced by cases detected by screening. *Int J Epidemiol* 1982b; 111:261–267.

Morrison AS: The author replies (letter to the editor). *Am J Epidemiol* 1983; 117:520.

Morrison AS: *Screening in Chronic Disease.* New York, Oxford University Press, 1985.

Morrison AS: Review of evidence on the early detection and treatment of breast cancer. *Cancer* 1989; 12(suppl):2651–2656.

Morrison AS: Is self-examination effective in screening for breast cancer? *J Natl Cancer Inst* 1991a; 83:226–227.

Morrison AS: Intermediate determinants of mortality in the evaluation of screening. *Int J Epidemiol* 1991b; 20:642–650.

Morrison AS, Brisson J, Khalid N: Breast cancer incidence and mortality in the Breast Cancer Detection Demonstration Project. *J Natl Cancer Inst* 1988; 80:1540–1547.

Moss S, Draper GJ, Hardcastle JD, Chamberlain J: Calculation of sample size in trials of screening for early diagnosis of disease. *Int J Epidemiol* 1987; 16:104–110.

Mulshine JL, Tockman MS, Smart CR: Considerations in the development of lung cancer screening tools. *JNCI* 1989; 81:900–906.

Multiple Risk Factor Intervention Trial Research Group: Mortality rates after 10.5 years for participants in the Multiple Risk Factor Intervention Trial. *JAMA* 1990; 263:1795–1801.

Multiple Risk Factor Intervention Trial Research Group: Multiple risk factor intervention trial: risk factor changes and mortality results. *JAMA* 1982; 248:1465–1477.

Murphy MFG, Campbell MJ, Goldblatt PO: Twenty years' screening for cancer of the uterine cervix in Great Britain, 1964–84: further evidence for its ineffectiveness. *J Epidemiol Comm Health* 1988; 42:49–53.

National Center for Health Statistics: Characteristics of females ever having a Pap smear and interval since last Pap smear, United States, 1973. *Monthly Vital Statistics Report* 1975; 24(7)(suppl):1–7.

Newcomb PA, Weiss NS, Storer BE, et al: Breast self-examination in relation to the occurrence of advanced breast cancer. *J Natl Cancer Inst* 1991; 83:260–265.

Olesen F: A case-control study of cervical cytology before diagnosis of cervical cancer in Denmark. *Int J Epidemiol* 1988; 17:501–508.

O'Malley MS, Fletcher SW: Screening for breast cancer with breast self-examination. A critical review. *JAMA* 1987; 257:2196–2203.

Oshima A, Hirata N, Ubukata T, et al: Evaluation of a mass screening program for stomach cancer with a case-control study design. *Int J Cancer* 1986; 38:829–833.

Ostrow JD, Discussant, in Brodie DR (ed): *Screening and Early Detection of Colorectal Cancer.* US Dept of Health, Education, and Welfare, National Cancer Institute, 1979, pp 167–170.

Palli D, Rosselli Del Turco M, Buiatti E, et al: A case-control study of the efficacy of a non-randomized breast cancer screening program in Florence (Italy). *Int J Cancer* 1986; 38:501–504.

Papanicolaou GN, Traut HF: *Diagnosis of Uterine Cancer by the Vaginal Smear.* New York, Commonwealth Fund, 1943.

Parkin DM, Nguyen-Dinh X, Day NE: The impact of screening on the incidence of cervical cancer in England and Wales. *Br J Obstet Gynaecol* 1985; 92:150–157.

Paul JR: Poliomyelitis immunization—1963. *Med Clin N Am* 1963; 47:1219–1230.

Peto R, Pike MC, Armitage O, et al: Design and analysis of randomized clinical trials requiring prolonged observation of each patient: I. Introduction and design. *Br J Cancer* 1976; 34:585–612.

Peto R, Pike MC, Armitage O, et al: Design and analysis of randomized clinical trials requiring prolonged observation of each patient: II. Analysis and examples. *Br J Cancer* 1977; 35:1–39.

Pettersson F, Bjorkholm E, Naslund I: Evaluation of screening for cervical cancer in Sweden: trends in incidence and mortality. *Int J Epidemiol* 1985; 14:521–527.

Pooling Project Research Group: Relationship of blood pressure, serum cholesterol, smoking habit, relative weight and ECG abnormalities to incidence of major coronary events: final report of the pooling project. *J Chron Dis* 1978; 31:201–306.

Powers CA: The work of the American Society for the control of cancer. *Medical Record* 1921; 99:211–213.

Prentice RL: A case-cohort design for epidemiologic studies and disease prevention trials. *Biometrika* 1986; 73:1–11.

Prentice RL: Surrogate endpoints in clinical trials: Definition and operational criteria. *Stat Med* 1989; 8:431–440.

Prorok PC: The theory of periodic screening: I. Lead time and proportion detected. *Adv Appl Prob* 1976a; 8:127–143.

Prorok PC: The theory of periodic screening: II. Doubly bounded recurrence times and mean lead time and detection probability estimation. *Adv Appl Prob* 1979b; 8:460–476.

Prorok PC, Hankey BF, Bundy BN: Concepts and problems in the evaluation of screening programs. *J Chron Dis* 1981; 34:159–171.

Roberts MM, Alexander FE, Anderson TJ, et al: Edinburgh trial of screening for breast cancer: mortality at seven years. *Lancet* 1990; i:241–246.

Robins JM: A new approach to causal inference in mortality studies with a sustained exposure period—application to control of the healthy worker survivor effect. *Mathematical Modelling* 1986; 7:1393–1512.

Robins JM: A graphical approach to the identification and estimation of causal parameters in mortality studies with sustained exposure periods. *J Chron Dis* 1987; 40:139s–161s.

Rogan WJ, Gladen B: Estimating prevalence from the results of a screening test. *Am J Epidemiol* 1978; 107:71–76.

Rose GA: CHD risk factors as a basis for screening, in Oliver M, Ashley-Miller M, Wood D (eds): *Screening for Risk of Coronary Heart Disease*. New York, Wiley, 1987, pp 11–14.

Rosenau MJ: *Preventive Medicine and Hygiene*, ed 2. New York, Appleton, 1927.

Rothman KJ: *Modern Epidemiology*. Boston, Little Brown & Co, 1986.

Rothman KJ, Boice JD Jr: *Epidemiologic Analysis with a Programmable Calculator*, US Dept of Health, Education, and Welfare, National Institutes of Health, 1979.

Saftlas AF, Szklo M: Mammographic parenchymal patterns and breast cancer risk. *Epidemiol Rev* 1987; 9:146–174.

Schlesselman JJ: *Case-control Studies: Design, Conduct, Analysis*. New York, Oxford University Press, 1982.

Selby JV, Friedman GD: Sigmoidoscopy in the periodic health examination of asymptomatic adults. *JAMA* 1989; 261:595–601.

Selby JV, Friedman GD, Collen MF: Sigmoidoscopy and mortality from colorectal cancer: the Kaiser Permanente Multiphasic Evaluation Study. *J Clin Epidemiol* 1988; 41:427–434.

Shapiro S, Strax P, Venet L: Periodic breast cancer screening: the first two years of screening. *Arch Environ Health* 1967; 15:547–553.

Shapiro S, Strax P, Venet L: Periodic breast cancer screening, in Sharp CLEH, Keen H (eds): *Presymptomatic Detection and Early Diagnosis*. London, Pitman, 1968; pp 203–236.

Shapiro S, Venet L, Strax P, et al: Ten- to fourteen-year effect of screening on breast cancer mortality. *JNCI* 1982; 69:349–355.

Shapiro S, Venet W, Strax P, Venet L: *Periodic Screening for Breast Cancer: The Health Insurance Plan Project and Its Sequelae, 1963–1986*. Baltimore, Johns Hopkins University Press, 1988.

Shaw GH: Use of Papanicolaou staining to predict urinary tract cancer. Paper presented at the State-of-the-Art Conference on Bladder Cancer Screening, Washington, DC, 1977.

Shwartz M: An analysis of the benefits of serial screening for breast cancer based upon a mathematical model of the disease. *Cancer* 1978; 41:1550–1564.

Shy K, Chu J, Mandelson M, et al: Papanicolaou smear screening interval and risk of cervical cancer. *Obstet Gynecol* 1989; 74:838–843.

Silverman DT, Morrison AS, Devesa SS: Bladder cancer, in Schottenfeld D, Fraumeni JF Jr (eds): *Cancer Epidemiology and Prevention*, ed 2. New York, Oxford University Press, 1992 (in press).

Silverstein M, Gamagami P, Colburn W, et al: Nonpalpable breast lesions: diagnosis with slightly overpenetrated screen-film mammography and hook wire-directed biopsy in 1,014 cases. *Radiology* 1989; 171:633–638.

Soini J, Hakama M: Failure of selective screening for breast cancer by combining risk factors. *Int J Cancer* 1978; 22:275–281.

Starreveld A, Hill GB, Brown LB, Koch M: Effect of screening on the incidence of cervical cancer in Alberta. *Canad Med Assoc J* 1981; 125:1105–1109.

Stevens GM, Weigen JF: Mammography survey for breast cancer detection. *Cancer* 1966; 19:51–59.

Stroehlein JR: Occult blood testing techniques and problems, in Brodie DR (ed): *Screening and Early Detection of Colorectal Cancer*, US Dept of Health, Education, and Welfare, National Cancer Institute, 1979, pp 153–157.

Tabar L, Fagerberg G, Duffy SW, Day NE: The Swedish two county trial of mammographic screening for breast cancer: recent results and calculation of benefit. *J Epidemiol Comm Health* 1989; 43:107–114.

Tabar L, Fagerberg CJG, Gad A, et al: Reduction in mortality from breast cancer after mass screening with mammography: randomized trial from the breast cancer screening working group of the Swedish National Board of Health and Welfare. *Lancet* 1985; i:829–832.

Task Force appointed by the Conference of Deputy Ministers of Health: Cervical cancer screening programs: The Walton Report. *Can Med Assoc J* 1976; 114:2–28.

Task Force to the Conference of Deputy Ministers of Health: *Periodic Health Examination Monograph*. Hull, Quebec, Canadian Government Publishing Centre, 1980.

Thorner RM, Remein QR: Principles and procedures in the evaluation of screening for disease. *Public Health Monogr* 1967; 67:1–24.

Tikkanen MJ, Nikkila EA: Current pharmacologic treatment of elevated serum cholesterol. *Circulation* 1987; 76:529–533.

UK Trial of Early Detection of Cancer Group: First results on mortality reduction in the UK trial of early detection of breast cancer. *Lancet* 1988; ii:411–416.

UK Trial of Early Detection of Cancer Group: Trial of early detection of breast cancer: description of method. *Br J Cancer* 1981; 44:618–627.

Van der Graaf Y, Zielhuis GA, Peer PGM, Vooijs PG: The effectiveness of cervical screening: a population-based case-control study. *J Clin Epidemiol* 1988b; 41:21–26.

Van der Graaf Y, Zielhuis GA, Vooijs GP: Cervical cancer mortality in the Netherlands. *Int J Epidemiol* 1988a; 17:270–276.

Vecchio TJ: Predictive value of a single diagnostic test in unselected populations. *N Engl J Med* 1966; 271:1171–1173.

Verbeek ALM, Hendriks JHCL, Holland R, et al: Reduction of breast cancer mortality through mass screening with modern mammography: first results of the Nijmegen project, 1975–1981. *Lancet* 1984; i:1222–1224.

Verbeek ALM, Hendriks JHCL, Holland R, et al: Mammographic screening and breast cancer mortality: age-specific effects in Nijmegen project, 1975–1982 (letter to the editor). *Lancet* 1985; i:865–866.

Veterans Administration Cooperative Study Group on Antihypertensive Agents: Effects of treatment on morbidity in hypertension: I. Results in patients with diastolic blood pressure averaging 115 through 129mm Hg. *JAMA* 1967; 202:1028–1034.

Veterans Administration Cooperative Study Group on Antihypertensive Agents: Effects of treatment on morbidity in hypertension: II. Results in patients with diastolic blood pressure averaging 90 through 114mm Hg. *JAMA* 1970; 213:1143–1152.

Veterans Administration Cooperative Study Group on Antihypertensive Agents: Effects of treatment on morbidity in hypertension: III. Influence of age, diastolic pressure, and prior cardiovascular disease; further analysis of side effects. *Circulation* 1972; 45:991–1004.

Wald NJ, Cuckle HS: Recent advances in screening for neural tube defects and Down's syndrome. *Bailliere's Clinical Obstetrics and Gynaecology* 1987; 1:649–676.

Walter SD, Day NE: Estimation of the duration of a pre-clinical disease state using screening data. *Am J Epidemiol* 1983; 118:865–886.

Walter SD, Stitt LW: Evaluating the survival of cancer cases detected by screening. *Stat Med* 1987; 6:885–900.

Wangsuphachart V, Thomas DB, Koetsawang A, Riotton G: Risk factors for invasive cervical cancer and reduction of risk by 'Pap' smears in Thai women. *Int J Epidemiol* 1987; 16:362–366.

Wechsler H, Levine S, Idelson RK, et al: The physician's role in health promotion—A survey of primary care practitioners. *N Engl J Med* 1983; 308:97–100.

Weinstein MC, Stason WB: *Hypertension: A Policy Perspective*. Cambridge, Mass, Harvard University Press, 1976.

Weiss NS: *Clinical Epidemiology: The Study of the Outcome of Illness*. New York, Oxford University Press, 1986.

Weiss NS: Control definition in case-control studies of the efficacy of screening and diagnostic testing. *Am J Epidemiol* 1983; 116:457–460.

Winawer SJ, Schottenfeld D, Flehinger BJ: Colorectal cancer screening. *JNCI* 1991; 83:243–251.

Wissler RW: The evolution of the atherosclerotic plaque and its complications, in Connor WE, Bristow JD (eds): *Coronary Heart Disease*. Philadelphia, Lippincott, 1985, pp 193–214.

Winslow CEA: *The Evolution and Significance of the Modern Public Health Campaign*. New Haven, Yale University Press, 1923, pp 57–61.

Witten DM, Thurber DL: Mammography as a routine screening examination for detecting breast cancer. *Am J Roentgenol Rad Therapy & Nuclear Med* 1964; 92:14–20.

Wolfe JN: Breast patterns as an index of risk for developing breast cancer. *Am J Roentgenol* 1976; 126:1130–1139.

Young JL Jr, Percy CL, Asire AJ (eds): Surveillance, Epidemiology, and End Results: Incidence and Mortality Data, 1973–77. *Natl Cancer Inst Monogr* 1981, 57:100.

Zelen M: Theory of early detection of breast cancer in the general population, in Heuson JC, Mattheim WH, Rozencweig M (eds): *Breast Cancer: Trends in Research and Treatment*. New York, Raven Press, 1976, pp 287–300.

Zelen M, Feinleib M: On the theory of screening for chronic diseases. *Biometrika* 1969; 56:601–614.

Index